30 Days of Sex Talks
Empowering Your Child with Knowledge of Sexual Intimacy
For Ages 12+

Educate and Empower Kids, LLC
© 2023 by Educate and Empower Kids

All rights reserved. Published 2023.

ISBN: 978-1-7367215-9-9

The paper used in this publication meets the minimum requirements of the American National Standard for Information Sciences— Permanence of Paper for Printed Library Materials, ANSI Z39.48-1992.

IF YOU ENJOYED THIS BOOK,
PLEASE LEAVE A POSITIVE REVIEW ON AMAZON.COM

Thank you to the following people for their support of our 30 Days of Sex Talks projects
Ed Allison
Mary Ann Benson, MSW, LSW
Scott Hounsell
Cliff Park

For great resources and information, follow us.

Facebook: www.facebook.com/lds.eduempowerkids
Twitter: @EduEmpowerKids
Pinterest: @EmpowerLDSKids
Instagram: @EduEmpowerKids
www.educateempowerkids.org

Be sure to check out our accompanying video series for this book at educateempowerkids.org

To view or download the additional resources listed at the end of each lesson, please follow the link in this QR code.

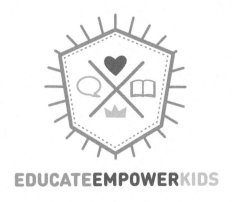

**EDUCATEEMPOWER**KIDS

Educate and Empower Kids would like to acknowledge the following people who contributed time, talents, and energy to this publication:

Dina Alexander, MS

Caron C. Andrews
K. Parker
Kaitlin Harker
Jenny Webb, MA
Amanda Scott

**Design and Illustration by:**
Jera Mehrdad and Zachary Hourigan

# 30 Days of

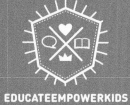

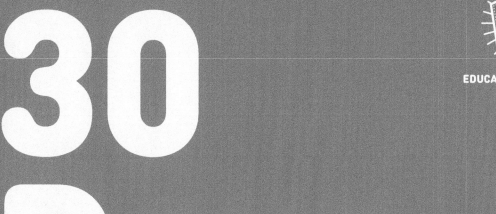

Sex

Talks

Empowering Your Child with
Knowledge of Sexual Intimacy

For AGES 12+

# 30 DAYS OF SEX TALKS
# TABLE OF CONTENTS

"I wholeheartedly believe that when we are fully engaged in parenting regardless of how imperfect, vulnerable, and messy it is, we are creating something sacred."

-BRENÉ BROWN

# INTRODUCTION

Dear Parents and Guardians,

Talking to our children about the powerful and significant nature of sexual intimacy is absolutely essential in our day. And the home is the perfect place to have these conversations with your children! We are living in complicated and uncertain times, and our kids are surrounded by unhealthy or false messages about their bodies, relationships, and human sexuality. It is our job to teach them what is true and what is not. It is vital that WE begin these discussions to help them understand what healthy sexuality is, how special their bodies are, AND that they can come to us as parents to find answers to questions.

Dieter Uchtdorf taught, "Since 'no other success can compensate for failure' here [in the home], we must place high priority on our families. We build deep and loving family relationships by doing simple things together, like family dinner and . . . by just having fun together. In family relationships love is really spelled t-i-m-e, time."

We also build deep and loving family relationships by having important, meaningful discussions! With these discussions, you have the opportunity to combat the negative messages our kids are hearing by sharing your wisdom, knowledge, and testimony about topics like love, healthy relationships, marriage, sexual intimacy, and the dangers that threaten their future happiness.

With this pragmatic, easy-to-use guide, we hope to provide you with an opportunity to start conversations about these essential topics. We also want to help you create a home environment which encourages open discussions about the many other issues which will inevitably come up as you raise your teen.

## WHAT'S INCLUDED

This curriculum includes helpful directions, 30 simple and invaluable lessons, and an extensive glossary of over 130 terms to help you. Each lesson includes introductory points to consider, critical teaching information, powerful discussion questions, and additional resources to enrich your family's learning experience. Some topics even have an accompanying activity or sample scenario to inspire further conversation.

## PREPARING FOR SUCCESS

- Plan ahead of time, but don't create an event. Having a plan or planning ahead of time will remove much of the awkwardness you might feel in talking about these subjects with your child. In not creating an event, you are making the discussions feel more spontaneous, the experience more repeatable, and yourself more approachable.

- Consider your individual child's age, developmental stage, and personality in conjunction with each topic, as well as your family's values and individual situation. These considerations will help you adapt the material in order to produce the best discussion. It's important that you begin your daily talks with just one topic in mind and that you make every experience, however brief, truly meaningful.

If you feel like your child isn't ready to discuss the bullets listed under the topic, or if you feel that your child's knowledge is more advanced, please note that we have also developed this curriculum for other age groups, and those curricula are available for purchase. It's important to discuss topics with your child based on their own maturity level and to progress through the curriculum or refer back to previous lessons at your own pace.

If you are positive and real with your child when it comes to talking about sexual intimacy, they will learn that you are available not just for this conversation, but for ANY discussion.

- Please know, you do not need to be an expert to have meaningful, informative discussions with your child. In fact, we feel strongly that leaning on your own personal experiences—both mistakes and successes—is a great way to use life lessons to teach your child. If done properly, these talks will bring you closer to your child than you could have ever imagined.

You know and love your child more than anyone, so you decide when and where these discussions take place. In time, you will recognize and enjoy teaching moments in everyday life with your child.

*Please know, you do not need to be an expert to have meaningful, informative discussions with your child.*

## NEED TO KNOW

- This program is meant to be simple! It's organized into simple topics with bullet points that are straightforward and create conversations. Each lesson may only take 10 minutes, but make sure you allow more time for your child's questions and extra family discussion.

- This curriculum is not a one-discussion-fits-all. You guide the conversation and lead the discussion according to your unique situation. If you have three children, you will likely have three different conversations about the same topic.

- No program can cover all aspects of sexual intimacy perfectly for every individual circumstance. You can empower yourself with the knowledge you gain from this program to share with your child what you feel is the most important.

# Create a Safe Zone

We recommend that you create a "safe zone" with your child and within your home. During the course of these conversations, your child should feel safe and free to ask any questions or make any comments without judgment or repercussions.

Your child should be able to use the term "safe zone" again and again to discuss, confide, and consult with you about the tough subjects they will be confronted with throughout life. It's highly recommended that, whenever possible, all parenting parties be involved in these discussions.

# INSTRUCTIONS
## ANSWER YOUR CHILD'S QUESTIONS

If you are embarrassed by your child's curiosity and questions, you're implying that there is something shameful about these topics. However, if you can answer their questions calmly and honestly, you're demonstrating that sexuality is positive and that healthy relationships are something to look forward to when the time is right. Be sure to answer your child's questions practically and cheerfully, and your child will learn that you are available not just for this discussion, but for any discussion. It's okay if you don't have all the answers, just tell them you will look for the answers and get back to them.

> **Taking the time to talk about these topics will reiterate to your child how important they are to you.**

## BE POSITIVE

Take the fear and shame out of these discussions. Sex is natural and wondrous, and your child should feel nothing but positivity about it from you. If you do feel awkward, stay calm and use matter-of-fact tones in your discussions. It's easier than you think—just open your mouth and begin! It will get easier with every talk you have. Even after just a few talks, both you and your child will begin to look forward to this time you are spending together. Use experiences from your own life to begin a discussion if it makes you feel more comfortable. We have listed some tough topics here, but they are all discussed in a positive, informative way. Don't worry, you've got this!

## FOCUS ON INTIMACY

Help your child understand how incredible and uniting sex can be. Don't just talk about the mechanics of sex. Spend a significant amount of time talking about the beauty of love and sex, the reality of human relationships, and the hows of building and maintaining those relationships. Children are constantly exposed to harmful examples of relationships in the media. Many of those examples are teaching your child misleading, incomplete, or purely unhealthy lessons about sexuality and interactions between people. Real emotional intimacy is rarely portrayed, so it's your job to teach and model what true intimacy actually is. Your child needs you to help connect the dots between healthy relationships and sexuality. Model positive ways for your child to care for and appreciate his or her body, as well as ways to protect, have a positive attitude toward, and make favorable choices for that body.

## BE THE SOURCE

Remember, you direct the conversations. Bring up the lesson points and questions that you feel are most important and allow the conversation to flow from there. You love and know your child better than anyone else, so you are the best person to judge what will be most effective. Pause and take into account your personal values, religious beliefs, individual personalities, and family dynamics. You can and should be the best source of information about sex and intimacy for your child. If you don't discuss these topics, your child will look for answers from other, less reliable, and sometimes harmful sources like the internet, various media, and other kids.

> You love and know your child better than anyone else, so you are the best person to judge what will be most effective.

Finally, throughout these conversations, you'll want to keep up a continuous, nonjudgmental dialogue about the topics in order to foster a healthy, open relationship with your child. Begin your daily talks with just one topic in mind and endeavor to make every experience, however brief, truly meaningful.

*Dina Alexander*
*Educate and Empower Kids*

# Let's Get Started!

Teenagers generally have more mature and complicated concerns about love, sex, and relationships, as well as how these topics connect with one another. Our program is meant to help you approach these subjects and facilitate meaningful dialogue, continuing to build on the solid foundation you've established. If you find yourself, like many, broaching these subjects with your child for the first time at this age, you will find helpful suggestions for how to get your child engaged in discussing their feelings and experiences. If you feel like your child needs more basic information before discussing the lessons and questions provided in this manual, refer back to the ages 8–11 curriculum.

Throughout these conversations, you'll want to keep up a continual, nonjudgmental dialogue about the topics provided. Remember, your child feels like they are adults, so respond as adult-like as possible.

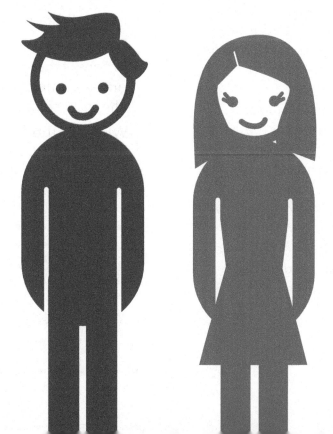

# 1.
# The Physical Side of Relationships

Dating and the physical side of dating relationships have evolved quite a bit in recent years. Take time to talk about dating etiquette, various forms of affection, and respect for oneself and for others.

Your son or daughter may feel various pressures from society, friends, or their partner to take a relationship to a sexual level. Help your teen set limits for themself now so that the decision need not be made in the heat of the moment. Also, help your teen come up with a plan to use if they get into a situation that is becoming too sexual for comfort. Make this plan very specific so that your teen won't get caught off guard in the middle of a situation with another person.

Ponder for yourself why teenagers are not emotionally or intellectually mature enough to handle serious dating relationships. Remember that one's brain has not finished developing until ages 22 to 24. This knowledge will help you communicate to your child why exclusive dating and certain levels of physical affection are usually big mistakes for teenagers.

## Start the Conversation

Talking about these issues will help teens identify and understand their own ideas and values about physical contact. Share your thoughts and beliefs, and perhaps even personal experiences of how you set and enforced your own limits when dating. You may consider pointing out prominent influences that helped shape your stance on physical affection.

## Questions for Your Child

- Q How might you know if you're ready to kiss someone?
- Q How might you know if someone is ready to kiss you?
- Q Where is the line between showing physical affection and turning that affection sexual?
- Q Which of the following shows affection? Examples are active listening, a gentle touch on the arm, smiling at each other, and/

**AFFECTION:** *A feeling of liking or caring for something or someone. A type of love that surpasses general goodwill.*

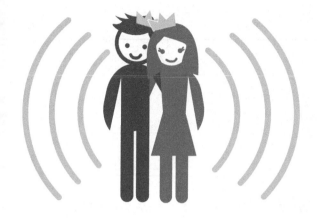

or maintaining eye contact. What other things show affection?

- Q If you get into a situation that is becoming too sexual for your comfort, what will you do and say? What will be your exit plan in that situation?

- Q Do societal concepts of sex come from biology?

- Q Are boys and girls born with certain inherent sexual urges and feelings?

- Q Are girls and boys socialized about sex in different ways?

- Q How do your family ideals about sex fit into your concept of sex?

- Q How does peer pressure factor into your concept of sex?

## Sample Scenario

Pose the following scenario to your teen to enhance the discussion and bring the subject into a real-life context:

You and your girlfriend have been getting physically closer the past few weeks with more intense kissing. You know you're on the edge of becoming sexually active with her. You've already decided how you feel about having sex—what circumstances will have to be in place and what you do/don't want to happen. Even so, you don't feel sure of what you want with her. Your girlfriend clearly feels sure about how she wants to proceed/ not proceed. How will you decide individually and as a couple what to do? What will you say to begin that conversation? Whose needs and wishes should prevail? How can you say no?

## Additional Resources:

"Helping Children Develop Healthy Sexual Attitudes" from Educate and Empower Kids
This article gives some helpful tools for parents on how to teach kids to develop healthier relationships with themselves and their growing sexualities.

"7 Questions to Help You Get Closer With Your Teenager" from Educate and Empower Kids
This article talks of a few different ways for us as parents to connect with our teenagers and show them that we truly care for them, their interests, and their lives.

"My Body Is Mine: Teaching Kids Appropriate Touch" from Educate and Empower Kids
This lesson is just as important for teenagers as it is for young children. Help your teen understand truly what is appropriate and inappropriate touch so that they may be empowered with knowledge that will help keep them safe throughout their lives.

# 2.
# Sex

You may think that you don't need to discuss the specifics of sex with your child, but the reality is that many teens are actively trying every kind of sex. Since your child is going to hear about sexual acts, you do need to explain certain aspects of sex with them. Initiating this conversation helps you be the source of information.

Even if you are uncomfortable talking about sex, it is important to talk about the various types (vaginal, anal, oral). Use the glossary to help you define these terms as well as other related terms, such as orgasm, ejaculation, erection, vagina, vulva, sex, vaginal secretions, etc.

## Start the Conversation

Ask your child how they define sex. Ask them what they think "counts" as sex. Various kinds of sex that were probably not discussed when you were a teenager are now part of everyday talk.

Steer the conversation toward the emotions and acceptability of the acts your child mentions. You can be a

powerful influence on how your teen feels about various forms of sexual contact and their personal decisions about them.

If you think there is even a small possibility that your child does not know how sex works, describe sexual intercourse. Here are some basics for sex between a man and a woman: A man places his erect penis into the vagina of his partner. She may help direct him to make insertion easier.

One or both partners may thrust rhythmically until the man or both of them orgasm. When he orgasms, sperm is released from his penis.

As you talk about sex to your children . . . remember to be frank, honest, and calm. Sex is an amazing, natural part of life and it's normal for your children to be curious about it.

> 📖 **INTERCOURSE:** *Sexual activity, also known as coitus or copulation, which is most commonly understood to refer to the insertion of the penis into the vagina (vaginal sex). It should be noted that there are a wide range of various sexual activities, and the boundaries of what constitutes sexual intercourse are still under debate.*

Often, a man helps his partner achieve orgasm before focusing on his orgasm. He helps his partner achieve orgasm by stimulating her genitals, especially her clitoris. As she feels more aroused, her vaginal area will become wet with vaginal secretions. This makes the insertion of the penis easier. With proper stimulation, the woman will orgasm. This can happen before the man places his penis into her vagina.

Let your child know that although simultaneous orgasm is usually portrayed in media, one partner often orgasms before the other. Discuss how this might be a better way to have intercourse, as it allows one person to focus on the pleasure of their partner and then have their partner focus their attention on them.

## Questions for Your Child

- ○ What do you think counts as sex? Is anything that results in an orgasm considered sex?

- ○ Is it sex if sex organs are touching but not orgasming? What if sex organs are not touching when orgasm is caused? Is having an orgasm sex if clothes are kept on?

- ○ What might be some of the consequences of having sex before you are ready?

- ○ What are the benefits of waiting to have sex until you are in a truly committed relationship or marriage?

---

## Additional Resources:

"Let's Talk About Sex: Talking to Teens & Tweens About Sex" from Educate and Empower Kids
This video goes through a few tactics on how to approach not only the subject of sex, but also how to navigate the various other sources that sexual information may come from (i.e., school, social media, their internet, etc.).

"8 Ways to Start Talking to Your Child About Sex" from Educate and Empower Kids
It can be difficult to talk to your child about sex, but it is a completely normal part of life. Read this article for more suggestions on how to talk to your child about sex.

# 3.
# Emotional Intimacy

Pop culture tends to portray sex as a purely selfish, physical interaction rather than an action based on a strong, healthy relationship. Help your child understand that sexual acts and emotional intimacy can be two separate things, but that they can often be more fulfilling when connected. Sex on its own can sometimes be an empty or selfish experience. The best sex often occurs in a committed relationship where both partners have real intimacy, mutual respect, and full confidence in their love.

Help your child understand what true intimacy is within a friendship AND a romantic relationship. Explain how lasting intimacy doesn't develop within a couple days. A deep friendship or romance takes time together, shared beliefs, genuine caring, and much more. The art of intimacy is a life-long pursuit.

## Start the Conversation
Discuss with your child what emotional intimacy includes: sharing feelings, ideas, dreams, experiences, and trust with another person.

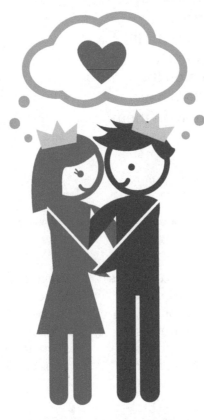

Emotionally intimate partners respect each other's differences and celebrate each other's uniqueness. They support and care for the other person as much as they care for themselves, or more. They truly want the best for that person.

Explain that physical sensations during sex are wonderful in and of themselves, but when they are combined with a deep, emotional connection, the experience involves much more than the physical enjoyment. It allows both partners to bond and become as one in a way that no other act can accomplish. Guide the conversation according to your experience and values, and be sure to also talk about why people may have sex for only the physical satisfaction.

Talk about how people sometimes confuse sex with true closeness or intimacy, when sex and intimacy can be two separate things depending on the emotions involved.

5

> 📖 **INTIMACY:** *Generally, a feeling or form of significant closeness. There are four types of intimacy: physical intimacy (sensual proximity or touching), emotional intimacy (close connection resulting from trust and love), cognitive or intellectual intimacy (resulting from honest exchange of thoughts and ideas), and experiential intimacy (a connection that occurs while working together). Emotional and physical intimacy are often associated with sexual relationships, while intellectual and experiential intimacy are not. However, people can engage in a sexual experience that is devoid of intimacy.*

## Questions for your Child

- ○ What do you think true intimacy is?
- ○ What do you think are the characteristics of a truly intimate friendship or romantic relationship?
- ○ Can you have a real romantic relationship without a physical relationship?
- ○ What behaviors and experiences can damage the emotional intimacy of a relationship?
- ○ How important is respect in a healthy sexual relationship?
- ○ How important is trust in a healthy sexual relationship?
- ○ How important is love in a healthy sexual relationship?
- ○ Can two people have a truly intimate relationship without having sex?
- ○ Why might the media rarely portray sex as needing true intimacy or marriage?

## Additional Resources:

"Intimacy Education Vs Sex Education" from Educate and Empower Kids
This article provides a perspective on how sex education goes beyond the physical aspects of the act. The article also encourages parents and guardians to put the topic of sex within the context of relationships and religion.

"Beyond the Sex Talks: Teaching Teens Emotional Intimacy" from Educate and Empower Kids
This article is a wonderful resource to teach teenagers and children about emotional intimacy and the importance of valuing themselves.

"10 Ways to Help Your Teen Take Back Their Emotions From Tech Distractions" from Educate and Empower Kids
This world is more and more tech-centered, and being so engrossed in technology has a negative impact on each of our emotions. This article goes through ten different tips on how to subvert that, especially for teens.

"Sex Ed Isn't Just for Kids" from Educate and Empower Kids
This article gives some advice on what Sex Ed should be and what kids and adults should understand about a healthy sex life.

# 4.
# Sex Means Different Things to Boys and Girls

Think about how the meaning of sexual intimacy has evolved over the past 100 years. What has our culture gained? What have we lost? What does sex mean to you? As you teach your child about the value and importance of sex, consider what you want your child to understand about how the world views sex versus how you view sex. Do you view sex as fun, special, mutually enjoyable, loving and/or passionate? Share your views.

## Start the Conversation

Due to differences in how boys and girls, or men and women, view sex, it's important that couples talk about it before engaging in it. Teach your child that open and honest communication will not lessen the romance; rather, it will enhance the relationship if couples understand the other's feelings, ideas, and concerns.

Ask your child what they think sex means to teenage boys and what they think sex means to teenage girls. Explain what you have learned over the years about the significance of sex. Then ask your child what they have learned about boys' and girls' perceptions of sex in the music they've heard, movies they've seen, and discussions they've listened to at school.

Then, discuss what you think sex means to people in a committed relationship. Remember that you are steering the conversation and can tailor it according to what you feel your child needs to hear the most.

## Questions for Your Child

○ How does the difference between boys' and girls' mindsets about sex affect the way they interact with members of the opposite gender?

○ What do you think are the biggest factors in determining the ideas that a boy has about sex? What are the factors that influence how a girl views sex?

**PERCEPTION:** *A way of regarding, understanding, or interpreting something; a mental impression.*

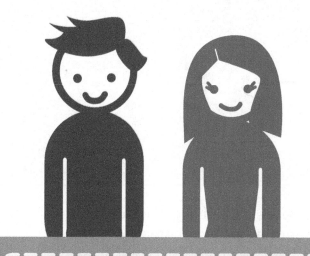

- Q Can you love someone romantically without it leading to sex?
- Q What do you think sex means to people in a committed relationship?
- Q How would you feel about a girl/boy who has sex for purely physical reasons?
- Q If your boyfriend or girlfriend wants to have sex with you, does that mean they love you?
- Q If you have the desire to have sex with a boyfriend or girlfriend, does that mean you love them?
- Q Are men and women really very different? How so? How are we similar?

> "Communication with your partner about the sexual aspect of your relationship is vital. As in any healthy relationship, good communication will help each of you in an intimate relationship understand the other and know each other's sexual feelings and expectations."
>
> -EDUCATE AND EMPOWER KIDS

## Additional Resources:

"Don't Have 'The Sex Talk' With Your Child—Have Many!" from Educate and Empower Kid
This article speaks to parents who are worried that they are too late to have the sex talk and reminds them that it is important to have many talks about sex with your children.

"8 Dangers of Sexting—and What Parents Can Do" from Educate and Empower Kids
In this article, we go through what sexting is, how damaging it is to all involved—especially when girls shoulder the blame for sending and boys do not for asking—and what we as parents can do about it.

"Is the Media Teaching Your Kids About Sex?" from Educate and Empower Kids
There are many ways in which sexual content in disguised as age-appropriate, especially with the prevalence of media and internet use now. This article lists a number of places where there is hidden sexual content for kids to find.

"8 Things Your Daughter Needs to Hear From YOU" from Educate and Empower Kids
"Whether we are talking about the birds and the bees, pornography and her developing brain, or her soon-to-arrive monthly visitor, there are things your daughter needs to know you know."

# 5.
# Positive Aspects of Sex

There are a lot of negative connotations about sex because, unfortunately, sex has been taught and practiced in inappropriate ways. Child molestation, rape, sexual abuse and pornography are gross misuses of sex. Also consider the negative tactic of "scaring" kids away from sex found in a lot of religious cultures. Though parents and community leaders generally hope to protect kids, the unintended side affect of this tactic is often that youth grow up feeling shameful, embarrased, or secretive about sex. However, you can counteract those negative influences by being warm and positive with your child when discussing sex.

Don't be afraid to talk about how sex can be an incredible, fun experience that feels great and fosters emotional bonding and unity between committed partners.

## Start the Conversation
Talk with your child about the unifying and bonding feelings that sex between loving, committed partners can create. Explain that sex is supposed to be pleasurable and satisfying under the right circumstances. Teach your teenager that creating life is an amazing, fantastic thing when emotionally and financially ready.

Explain how during sex the body releases endorphins (reducing anxiety and stress), dopamine (engaging the brain's reward system and making us feel good), and oxytocin (causing feelings of emotional bonding, loyalty, and trust). Discuss how the release of these hormones and molecules can deeply impact how we feel about a person when we have sex with them.

**HEALTHY SEXUALITY:**
*Having the ability to express one's sexuality in ways that contribute positively to one's own self-esteem and relationships. Healthy sexuality includes approaching sexual relationships and interactions with mutual agreement and dignity. It necessarily includes mutual respect and a lack of fear, shame, or guilt, and it never includes coercion or violence.*

Emphasize that a healthy outcome of connecting physically is connecting emotionally on a very intimate and human level. Intense and vulnerable feelings naturally flow from healthy sex between people who love and deeply care for one another. This is the amazing and bonding aspect that makes sex very special and personal to a married couple. Sex is meant to unify two people in this way. It is meant to be good.

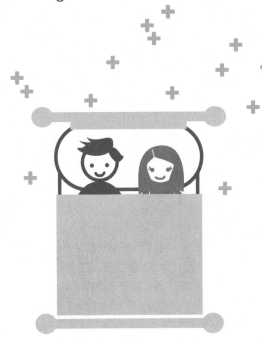

## Questions for Your Child

- ☮ What positive things have you heard about sex?

- ☮ What do you think would make sex a very positive experience? Does it include emotional closeness and trust? Does it include chemistry between you and your partner?

- ☮ Are the physical feelings associated with sex as pleasurable as the emotional?

- ☮ Can you have a positive experience with hook-up sex?

- ☮ Sex often makes us feel bonded, attached, and deeply connected. Should these feelings be saved for a committed relationship or is it okay to share these with a person we are casually dating?

## Additional Resources:

"Did I Wait Too Long? Starting the Sex Talk With an Older Teen" from Educate and Empower Kids
This article offers tips for getting the conversation started with older kids and how to keep that conversation going.

"4 Easy Steps to Develop Unhealthy Sexuality" from Educate and Empower Kids
This article satirically lists things you can do as parents to instill bad habits and unhealthy ways of thinking in your kids. Ultimately it shows what not to do and not to teach to raise mentally healthy children.

"Talking With Your Teen About Sex" from Educate and Empower Kids
This article includes pointers and definitions about sexual terms and how to talk to your teenager about sex.

"Does Talking About Pornography With Your Kids 'Give Them Ideas'?" from Educate and Empower Kids
This article talks about the importance of giving information and being that source of information for your kids.

# 6.
# Physical Responses to Sex

Your personal comfort level and dynamics with your teenager will naturally dictate how you approach this topic. Guide this conversation according to your values and beliefs about the nature of sex. Our goal is to help you educate your child about the positive physical reactions to sex, about how wonderful they can be under the right circumstances, and about possible negative physical reactions. Knowing that there is a range of responses from healthy to problematic can help your child understand themselves, their future partner, and healthy sexuality. Be sure to include your personal views and family expectations in the conversation.

## Start the Conversation

According to your comfort level, explain the physical progression of arousal. See the glossary for definitions of unfamiliar words. When explaining these responses, remind your child that physical responses are individual and vary from person to person.

When a female is aroused, the nipples and external genitals—including the labia and clitoris—become engorged. There is vaginal lubrication and secretions, which aid in physically comfortable intercourse. The vagina enlarges with arousal. When a woman orgasms, she experiences intense feelings of pleasure and the muscles of her vagina may rhythmically spasm. She may also experience one or more orgasms following her first.

When a male is stimulated, blood flow to the penis increases, causing an erection. During this process, the skin of the scrotum tightens and the testicles are pulled in close to the body. The head of the penis typically enlarges with the influx of blood. Prior to ejaculation, some fluid may be released from the tip of the penis. At the climax of sexual excitement, or orgasm, ejaculation occurs.

**AROUSAL:** *The physical and emotional response to sexual desire during or in anticipation of sexual activity. In men, this results in an erection. In women, vaginal lubrication (wetness), engorgement of the external genitals (clitoris and labia), and enlargement of the vagina.*

11

Not all male erections are due to sexual arousal. Talk about spontaneous erections, which can occur when awake or asleep for physiological, nonsexual reasons.

You may want to also discuss specific sexual problems that can occur. Some include priapism (see glossary), which is a male's prolonged erection; vaginismus (see glossary), which is the inability to penetrate vaginally; female vaginal dryness, which can make intercourse uncomfortable or painful; and erectile dysfunction, which is the male's inability to achieve or keep an erection. Note that the growing rate of erectile dysfunction in the male population is linked to prolonged exposure to and use of online pornography (Voon, et al., 2014). You may want to talk about this with your child both now and when you discuss pornography in lesson #17.

## Questions for Your Child

Q It is quite natural to become aroused by something on TV, an attractive person, etc., but we usually can't act on these feelings immediately. What is a positive way to channel that energy elsewhere?

Q Does arousal being a natural force make it okay to act on? Should sexual arousal be controlled?

Q When dating or spending time with people we are attracted to, is there a way to avoid getting too aroused?

Q Why is sexual arousal so powerful?

Q Can you be aroused without having a sexual experience?

---

"As parents, we should want our children to grow up to experience fulfilling and satisfying sexuality ... creating open dialogues in your home will help your child to not only develop healthy sexual attitudes, but have a satisfying sex life based in intimacy and connection."

-EDUCATE AND EMPOWER KIDS

---

## Additional Resources:

"Helping Children Develop Healthy Sexual Attitudes" from Educate and Empower Kids
This article is a resource meant to help parents talk about sexuality with their children. It provides helpful tips and pointers as parents talk about arousal and other common feelings.

"4 Easy Steps to Creating Healthy Communication About Sexual Intimacy" from Educate and Empower Kids
This article will help you and your children create healthy communication habits that will make the sex talks easier.

# 7.
# Orgasm

Orgasm is a natural part of sex. It's a huge topic of conversation and a focal point in pornography, which has filtered down through the mainstream, making orgasm's importance somewhat inflated and exaggerated. Teenagers need to understand what orgasm is, what it's for, and how its presence or absence can affect an intimate sexual relationship. If you are comfortable, discuss with your teen the different ways of achieving an orgasm and the potential for multiple orgasms. Explain that men and women achieve orgasm differently.

For centuries, female pleasure and female orgasm have not been considered important or even acceptable. Teach your daughter that her sexual experience is just as important as her partner's. Talk to your daughter about how she can achieve orgasm. Discuss clitoral stimulation and other erogenous zones. It is also important to teach your son that both sexual partners help each other achieve orgasm.

Help your child understand that simultaneous orgasm (as portrayed in television and pornography) is often not accurate, nor is it necessarily more pleasurable than each person having their orgasm individually. Explain how it might be beneficial for one person to focus on the pleasure of their partner and then their partner to reciprocate that attention.

*See the glossary for helpful definitions, such as clitoris, erection, ejaculation, vagina, nocturnal emissions, and more.

 **ORGASM:** *The rhythmic muscular contractions in the pelvic region that occur as a result of sexual stimulation during the sexual response cycle. Orgasms are characterized by a sudden release of built-up sexual tension and by the resulting sexual pleasure.*

## Start the Conversation

Explain the differences between female and male orgasm. Female orgasm is frequently achieved as a result of the physical, sexual stimulation of the clitoris (and/or through vaginal penetration for 18% of women). Female orgasm results in a release of the buildup of sexual tension and excitement through involuntary spasms of the pelvic area and vagina. It is accompanied by a general euphoric and intensely pleasurable physical sensation and can include spontaneous vocalizations.

Males generally reach orgasm through physical, sexual stimulation of the penis, beginning with getting an erection. At the point of climax, sexual tension and excitement typically culminate in ejaculation and involuntary spasms in the pelvic area. As with female orgasm, it is accompanied by a general euphoric and intensely pleasurable physical sensation and can include spontaneous vocalizations.

Discuss the normality of nocturnal emissions, which are orgasms in either males or females that occur spontaneously during sleep. A common expression for them in males is "wet dreams." Have a discussion about epididymal hypertension (see glossary), commonly called "blue balls," which occurs when fluid temporarily overfills

the testicles because of prolonged and unfulfilled sexual arousal. It can cause pain or discomfort in the testicles. However, though epididymal hypertension may be uncomfortable, remind your daughter that she is not obligated to complete a sexual act once begun in order to avoid the man's discomfort. Either partner can stop the sexual experience at any time.

Finally, it is critical to teach your child that they must express their sexual needs to their partner. This seems to be more difficult for women, as many are not taught that their sexual needs are important.

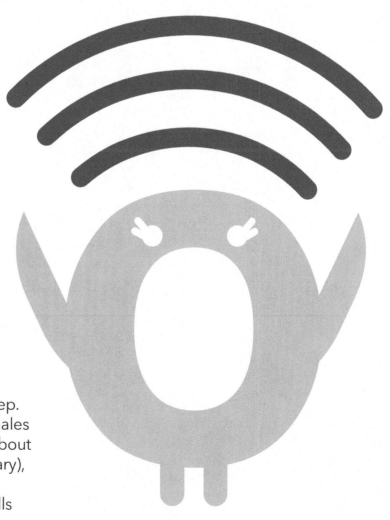

# "Sex is about the quality of your entire love life, not the intricate alignment of your bodies."

## -KEVIN LEMAN

## Questions for Your Child

- How does orgasm differ for males and females?

- Is having an orgasm the most important factor in sex? Why might other aspects of sex be just as important?

- Can sex still be fulfilling even if you don't orgasm?

- If orgasm is not achieved, is it something to feel bad about?

- Do most couple's orgasms happen at the same time (as portrayed in TV and movies)?

- Are you obligated to complete a sexual act once begun in order to avoid your sexual partner's discomfort? (The absolute, irrevocable answer to this is no.)

- Sex is an amazing experience. Why might it be a good idea to wait until you are in a committed relationship to have sex?

- The world often depicts sex as something that you do TO someone. Done the right way, sexual intimacy is something you experience together. What is the difference?

- What other questions do you have about orgasms?

## Additional Resources:

"Common Mistakes Parents Make When Talking To Kids About Sex" from Educate and Empower Kids
This article points out four common mistakes that parents make when it comes to opening the door for healthy conversations about sex and body image.

"Common Questions Kids Ask About Sex (And How to Answer)" from Educate and Empower Kids
This article covers some of the most common questions that kids have about sex and intimacy (including orgasm) and how to answer them confidently.

# 8.
# Relationship Boundaries

Many teenagers do not know what boundaries are or how to enforce their personal boundaries. However, boundaries serve as an important part of any healthy relationship. That is why it is imperative that you teach your child what boundaries are and how to create healthy boundaries for themself. Boundaries establish needed space between your child and another person. Boundaries are the spoken or unspoken rules of how your child will treat someone and how they expect to be treated.

When healthy boundaries are not established, the relationship and the people involved suffer. Boundaries help us communicate respect and love by allowing us to express ourselves, our wants, desires, beliefs, likes, and dislikes. Sharing these things with those we care about helps create mutual respect within the relationship and allows space for growth.

Our book *30 Days to a Stronger Child* has great family night discussions to help you talk about boundaries, assertiveness, respect, friendship, accountability, empathy, and other topics related to our intellectual, physical, social, spiritual and emotional "accounts."

## Start the Conversation

This discussion continues some of the points from the first topic of this book, "The Physical Side of Relationships." Encourage your child to make a decision about their boundaries and standards before they are in a sexual situation. Talk about other standards a person should have in place before the situation arises such as for cheating in class, trying drugs, posting certain things on social media, etc. Explain that the older we are, the more sure we are of our physical and emotional boundaries, and the more capable we are of being true to those personal boundaries.

**BOUNDARIES:** *The personal limits or guidelines that an individual forms in order to clearly identify what are reasonable and safe behaviors for others to engage in around him or her.*

Explain and make sure your teen understands that they never have to kiss, hug, touch, or have sex with anyone they don't want to. The objective here is for your teen to know that they are in charge of their bodies, and that they can decide what physical and emotional affection they are comfortable with.

## Questions for Your Child

○ What are some examples of healthy physical and emotional boundaries you have with your friends? What about with those you are dating?

○ What are some examples of unhealthy boundaries? (Calling or texting too much, demanding too much time, asking invasive questions, pushing someone to have sex, pressuring someone to go against their own beliefs, etc.)

○ What can you do when friends, boyfriends/girlfriends, classmates, etc. overstep their boundaries? How do you uphold your personal beliefs and standards with friends and others?

○ What boundaries do your parents have with their friends, with people in the neighborhood or at work, or with you?

○ What role does self-respect play in setting your boundaries?

○ Our instincts and our personal "conscience" can help us know our personal boundaries. How can you learn to listen to your inner voice and your instincts?

○ If your partner wants to have sex but you don't, how will you put a limit or boundary on certain physical contact?

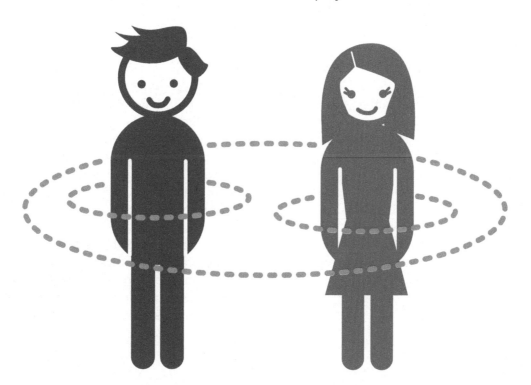

## Sample Scenario

Pose the following scenario to your teen to enhance the discussion and bring the subject into a real-life context:

> Your best friend comes to you for advice on what to do with a person they're very attracted to that has made it clear they'd be up for a sexual hookup. You know that having sex before being in a committed relationship is a huge mistake. What will you say to your friend? What kinds of questions could you ask them to help them come to a decision that they feel is right?

## Additional Resources:

"Lesson: Teaching Your Kids Healthy Boundaries" from Educate and Empower Kids
This family lesson offers a guided approach to teaching your kids about building and maintaining healthy boundaries.

"Creating Rules and Boundaries With Your Family" from Educate and Empower Kids
This article provides a definition of boundaries and lays out how you can implement them in your family.

"Text-Dominant Relationships: A Social Norm that Is Killing Meaningful Teen Relationships" from Educate and Empower Kids
"A deeper sense of empathy and emotional connection can only be nurtured face to face and are needed to build strong and loving relationships."

"For Parents: How to Have a Family Council" from Educate and Empower Kids
This lesson goes through ways to have a meaningful and uplifting family council, where you will be able to connect and communicate.

When healthy boundaries are not established, the relationship, as well as those involved, suffer. Boundaries help us to communicate respect and love by allowing us to express ourselves.

# 9.
# The First Time

Most teenagers and many college-age adults feel unprepared for their first sexual experience. According to what you know of your teen, share your wisdom. Help them understand how this is the most vulnerable and sensitive experience they may ever have and why it is so important to choose a partner wisely. Explain that their first time will most likely go more smoothly and be more meaningful if their partner is someone who loves them and cares deeply for them. If you believe in waiting to have sex until you are in a committed relationship or marriage, explain why.

Have a discussion about how having sex adds a new dimension to an already close relationship. Help your teen develop a sense of how special and unifying sexual intimacy can be. Emphasize that they can decide beforehand the circumstances they will require for their first time. Discuss what it means to be ready for a sexual relationship (emotionally, spiritually, intellectually, and physically).

*Helpful terms in the glossary include intimacy, hymen, premature ejaculation, vaginal sex, and vaginal discharge/secretions.

## Start the Conversation

Without going into graphic detail, tell your child what some of your fears or expectations were about sex before you actually had your first experience. Ask your teen what expectations they have for their first time. Do they expect everything to go smoothly? What kind of birth control will they use?

Reiterate your family values and personal thoughts on when it is appropriate to have sex for the first time. If your family is religious, feel free to share these views as well. Talk about the emotional impact of a sexual relationship. Discuss that some girls/women experience slight pain (or a lot of pain) with their first intercourse due to the tightening of vaginal muscles or the stretching or breaking of the hymen (see glossary). Have a discussion about

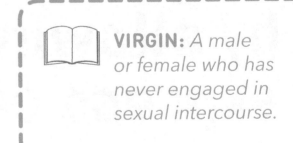

**VIRGIN:** *A male or female who has never engaged in sexual intercourse.*

how having sex changes a relationship. Help your teen develop a sense of sex as a special bond between two people.

Discuss what attitude will be helpful if the first experience doesn't go exactly to plan. Talk about premature ejaculation (see glossary) and how it can impact a sexual experience physically and emotionally. Discuss the myth that a girl can't get pregnant the first time and the importance of birth control. More information on birth control can be found under "Birth Control" (lesson #30).

## Questions for Your Child

Q Is it okay to have sex for the first time if you are in love and in a committed relationship?

Q When you imagine your ideal first time, are you married?

Q Is the ideal situation for your first time being in a solid, committed relationship? Is the ideal situation being with a sexy stranger with whom sparks are flying?

Q Is sex usually enjoyable the first time for both people? Is there ever pain or discomfort?

Q Can a relationship ever go back to what it was before having sex?

Q What do you think might be some negative changes in a relationship once you've started having sex?

Q What do you think might be some positive changes in a relationship once you've started having sex?

Q What if after your first time, you don't like it? Will it always be that way? How should you talk about it with your partner?

Communication with our kids gives them an avenue for releasing stress and receiving advice, and it also provides a sounding board for them. Sometimes we simply need to bounce ideas and thoughts off of someone. Parents, we can provide these things for our kids if we practice open communication! If we don't, we can be sure they will find this stress relief, advice, and sounding board in other people, potentially people who will give them wrong ideas and even dangerous advice.

## Additional Resources:

"Five Great Ways to Bring Truly Open Communication to Your Home" from Educate and Empower Kids
Communication is a crucial part of parenting, and this article provides ways to improve communication with your children.

"How to Overcome the Trepidition of Talking to Your Kids About Sex" from Educate and Empower Kids
This video goes over a few points on how to have those scary sex talks with your kids and how to ease any anxiety to reduce that fear or apprehension.

# 10.
# Consent

It would be nice if we could assume that our children will always be safe or that they won't even think about sex until they are engaged to be married. But this just isn't a reality for many teens and young adults. So we must prepare our girls AND boys to respect themselves and others physically, intellectually and emotionally. Our teens must understand both for themselves and for others what constitutes consent when it comes to kissing, other physical affection, and sexual intercourse. Then they will know when yes really means yes.

 **CONSENT:** *Clear agreement or permission to permit something or to do something. Consent must be given freely, without force or intimidation and while the person is fully conscious and cognizant of their present situation.*

Take time to have a meaningful discussion about the types of things that make up rape culture, such as blaming the victim, making jokes about rape, watching gendered violence in movies, assuming that only promiscuous women—and never men—get raped, and tolerating sexual harassment. When teaching this lesson, keep in mind that rape and harrasment happen to girls AND boys.

*See the glossary for definitions of test touch, rape, rape culture, and sexual harassment.

## Start the Conversation

Explain to your child what consent is. There's an old notion (often portrayed in pornography) that when a woman says "no," she really means yes. Discuss this notion and possible reasons for it with your teen. If you find that your child has bought into the idea that no really means yes, emphatically set them straight. Having sex with someone without their consent is forcible or coerced rape. Ask your teen if they fully understand what rape is.

Discuss how to stay safe in various situations. Come up with a plan! Being

grabbed, pinched, or touched in any way that's not wanted or comfortable is never okay. If it's unwanted, it needs to stop. Emphasize that your child should expect to be treated with respect and dignity everywhere.

If anyone touches your teen in a way that they don't consent to, it needs to be immediately stopped so that it doesn't progress. This kind of touching can start with a "test touch," such as a touch to the arm or a hug. It can then progress further to the point that the touch is uncomfortable and unwanted. Tell your teenager that even if they liked hugging or other physical contact with someone before, they can stop it if it becomes uncomfortable or more than what they want. Consent is also discussed in lesson #23, "Unwanted Sexual Attention."

## Questions for Your Child

○ Sexual harassment is fairly prevalent in high school and even middle school. What have you observed in your schools?

○ If a person does not respect another's "no," when does it become harassment?

○ Besides sex, what are some other forms of physical affection where you should give or receive consent before proceeding?

○ What is rape? What is rape culture?

○ How will you know your partner is giving clear consent to have sex?

○ What can you say and do if you are being pressured to have sex?

○ Is it okay to stop sex or physical affection once you've started?

Q How does good communication relate to determining what your partner truly wants?

Q If a person is using drugs or alcohol, how does that affect the ability to give true consent? What else could make it difficult to give true consent?

## Sample Scenario

Pose the following scenario to your teen:

Samantha is at a party and has had two beers. She usually doesn't drink, and she's feeling a bit light-headed. Everything seems silly to her. She is flirting back and forth with a guy she knows but has never really noticed before. She feels silly and giddy, and this boy suddenly seems to her like the greatest person in the room. He has also had a few drinks and starts making sexual overtures toward Samantha. She feels so tipsy that sex with him seems like a good idea. They find a secluded spot together.

## Ask the following questions:

Q If Samantha has sex with the boy, has Samantha truly given consent? Has the boy? Do you think this would play out differently if one or both of them weren't impaired by alcohol?

## Additional Resources:

Lesson: Talking to Your Kids About Consent from Educate and Empower Kids
This lesson teaches about the importance of not giving into unwanted attention and ensuring that everyone receives respect.

"Consent: Not Actually That Complicated (Clean Edition!)" from Educate and Empower Kids
This article breaks down just how simple consent really is by using the analogy of making someone a cup of tea.

"Peer on Peer Abuse: Why It Happens and What Parents Can Do" from Educate and Empower Kids
In this video, the reasons for peer-on-peer abuse are discussed along with solutions on how to stop this before it becomes a problem.

Teach your child
that they have the
power to say

# "NO!"

Empower them
by teaching that
if someone is being
physical with them
in a way
they do not like,
they can say no
& get away.
They have that
right & power.

# 11.
# Creating a Healthy Relationship

Healthy relationships in all areas of our lives are important to our happiness and sense of well-being. They're also the basis of positive, healthy sexual experiences. The hypersexualized and porn-influenced culture that kids are steeped in doesn't teach about true intimacy, kindness, emotional health, or solid, committed relationships.

> Teaching children how to build healthy relationships will enable them to recognize when a relationship is unhealthy, create healthy relationships, and help others foster healthy relationships.

Explain some of the aspects of developing a healthy relationship: learning to communicate well, cultivating respect and dignity, developing healthy ideas of intimacy, and getting to know someone over time. Discuss the need for a relationship to move beyond infatuation in order to mature into a truly healthy relationship. Share your opinion on how long a couple should date and get to know each other before they are ready to get married.

## Start the Conversation

Discuss your vision and hope for the kind of committed relationship your child will have when they are adults. Point out examples of healthy relationships in your teen's life. Teach your teen that both people in a relationship deserve respect and dignity and that no two people are going to agree 100% of the time. Discuss what good communication looks and sounds like in a healthy relationship (kind words, respect for others' opinions, listening to the other person, expressing oneself clearly, etc.).

Ask your child what kind of person they would like to marry someday. What type of personality might their spouse have? What things might they both have in common? What are the top five most important traits for their spouse to possess?

Explain that teenage years are for learning about relationships with the hope of learning what true intimacy is. Part of true intimacy is learning how to disagree and that disagreements are okay. Talk about what is appropriate etiquette when discussing differences, such as not calling names and not bringing up past arguments. Power struggles within a relationship can make one person feel inferior to the other. Talk with your teen about how power struggles can be diminished when each person has a healthy sense of self, as well as respect for self and partner.

## Questions for Your Child

- Q How do you know whether your relationships with others are healthy or unhealthy?

- Q What can you do to improve your relationship with your parents? With your siblings? With friends and classmates?

- Q What kind of behaviors, language, and actions does a healthy relationship include?

- Q Is a healthy relationship a "perfect" relationship?

- Q How does each person in a healthy relationship keep their own individuality yet still remain united?

- Q How do you like to communicate your feelings, thoughts, and desires?

- Q How can you be clear in your communication without putting another person down?

- Q What can you do to end a relationship that is not healthy?

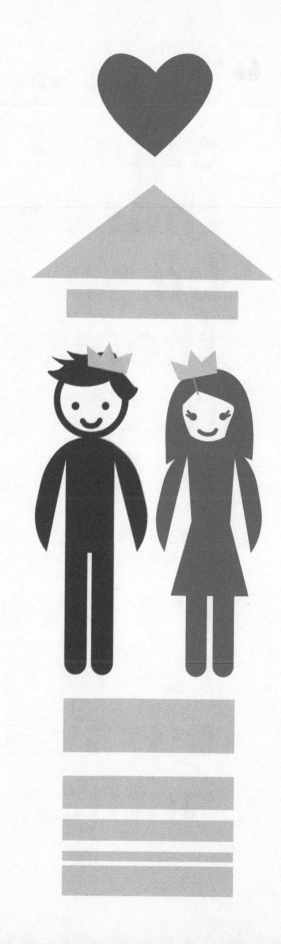

**"The beginning of love is to let those we love be perfectly themselves, and not to twist them to fit our own image. Otherwise we love only the reflection of ourselves we find in them."**

-THOMAS MERTON

## Activity

Write each of the bulleted points on separate pieces of paper. Pass one or two pieces of paper to each member of your family. Have each person take a turn reading their paper and giving examples of how their points are important to healthy relationships. Share your wisdom and encourage everyone to add their ideas or questions to the conversation.

- Respect for each other's agency, autonomy, and boundaries
- Honesty and trust
- Compromising to meet each other's needs
- Open communication of thoughts and feelings
- Honoring differences and strengths
- Sharing similar values and beliefs
- Responsibility and accountability

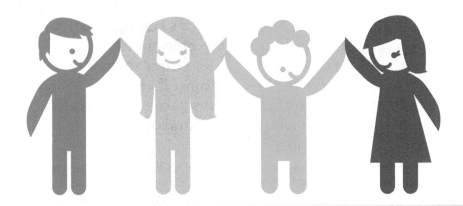

## Additional Resources:

"Preparing Our Kids for Courtship in the Digital Age" from Educate and Empower Kids
It is important for our children to know the different aspects of a relationship and how one develops a relationship.

"How to Create Healthy Relationships" from Educate and Empower Kids
This family lesson is a great place to start in discussing how to create and develop healthy relationships. It also speaks about the importance of having and maintaining those healthy relationships.

"Kids in the Digital Age: The Challenge of Expressing Emotions Healthily" from Educate and Empower Kids
As children learn to express their emotions healthily, they will be learning how to create better and healthier relationships.

"Kids and Dating in the Digital Age" from Educate and Empower Kids
This video goes through a few of the challenges of dating in the digital age and ways to help kids figure out how to navigate it all.

"6 Great Activities to Help You Communicate With Your Teenager" from Educate and Empower Kids
With the knowledge that communication is the key to all healthy relationships, this article goes through a few ways to improve your communication with your teenager.

# 12.
# Abusive Relationships

Everyone deserves relationships that are free from fear and abuse. Abuse can be anything from persistent verbal bullying all the way to physical violence. Be sure your teen understands that abuse can be emotional, mental, physical, and/or sexual. You may find this "Power and Control Wheel" graphic from the National Domestic Violence Hotline useful for identifying abusive behaviors. Remind your child that although most people are good and kind, your child will know abusive people in their life.

This is also a great time to talk about why it's so important for your kid to develop their own interests and talents, build their sense of self-worth, and treat themself kindly. The stronger they are in these areas, the less likely they will be vulnerable to abuse.

## Start the Conversation

Discuss what abusive relationships and domestic violence are (see glossary). The United States Department of Justice defines domestic violence as "a pattern of abusive behavior in any relationship that is used by one partner to gain or maintain power and control over another intimate partner. Domestic violence can be physical, sexual, emotional, economic, or psychological actions or threats of actions that influence another person. This includes any behaviors that intimidate, manipulate, humiliate, isolate, frighten, terrorize, coerce, threaten, blame, hurt, injure, or wound someone."

**DOMESTIC ABUSE/ DOMESTIC VIOLENCE:** *A pattern of abusive behavior in any relationship that is used by one partner to gain and/or maintain power and control over another in a domestic setting. It can be physical, sexual, emotional, economic, and/ or psychological actions or threats of actions that harm another person.*

Help your child understand that abusers do not start out abusing right away, and they can often be attractive, charming, and other great qualities. Teach your teen to trust their gut instinct when something doesn't feel right instead of waiting for something bad to happen.

Teach your teen that it's not okay to call names or allow anyone to speak to them in a way they find disrespectful. This is often where a pattern of poor behavior or abuse begins. It's also not okay for anyone to put their hands on your child in a way your child doesn't like. Repeated exposure to this kind of treatment desensitizes the victim, and they may not easily identify escalating abuse.

Talk about what a person can do to get help out of an abusive relationship and stop the cycle. Telling others about the abuse is a key step. It can sometimes be hard to identify abuse in dating relationships because of the emotions involved. Emphasize that there are people your teen can talk to, such as their counselors at school and you as their parent or guardian. There are also help centers and hotlines that are easily accessible online.

## Questions for Your Child

- ○ What is physical abuse? Verbal abuse? Sexual abuse? Emotional abuse?

- ○ Think carefully. Do you ever say or do things that could be considered abusive?

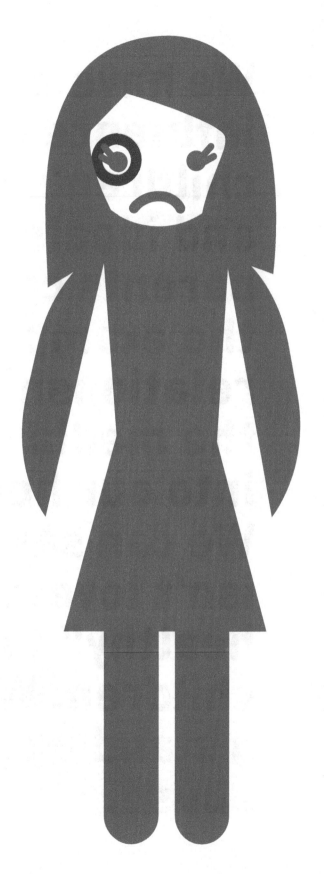

We have a powerful influence on our children's standards and ideals. We as parents can set the example in our relationships and in the media we bring into our homes. We can say "this isn't love; this isn't healthy" to our children. We can take a stand against abuse.

- Has anyone ever abused you?

- What can you do now to ensure that you will never be abusive toward others in your words or actions?

- Have you ever seen an abusive relationship? What does it look like? How do the people involved behave?

- How is power and control at the heart of abusive behavior?

- How can a person who has been abused as a child grow up to have healthy relationships?

- How can you identify abusive people and situations? What can you do to end a relationship that is not healthy?

## Sample Scenario

Pose the following scenario to your teen. You and a classmate are becoming good friends. They have been teasing you about a birthmark you have on your arm that you initially joked about. Lately though, their comments and jokes are making you uncomfortable, self-conscious, and mad.

## Ask the following questions:

- How will you handle this? What reaction might you receive if you snap at them and walk away?

- Will you just stop laughing along with them and hope they take a hint?

- How might you say something to them directly the next time it happens?

- What does this scenario have to do with healthy or abusive relationships?

## Additional Resources:

National Domestic Violence Hotline
This is a web page with numerous resources available, including great definitions and explanations for abuse that occurs in dating and other relationships.

"The Fifty Shades Effect: Disempowerment of Young Girls and What We Can Do About It" from Educate and Empower Kids
This article talks of the different damaging messages portrayed in Hollywood and in movies our kids might view, as well as countermeasures against those messages.

"Real Life Lessons Learned From Beauty and the Beast" from Educate and Empower Kids
This helpful article discusses counterfeit messages our kids receive about relationships and how to combat their ill effects.

"Online Bullying: What to Do!" from Educate and Empower Kids
"As parents, this is something we must have on our radar, as it is likely our child will either be the victim of cyberbullying, have a friend who is being bullied, or be a bully themselves."

# 13.
# Self Worth & Sex

The term "self-esteem" has been overused in so many ways that truly understanding self-worth has become difficult for many. In the past 50 years, people have been encouraged to "love" themselves in order to truly love others. But most people don't actually love themselves. However, most people can take care of their own emotional needs

 **SELF-ESTEEM/SELF-WORTH:** *An individual's overall emotional evaluation of their own worth. Self-esteem is both a judgment of the self and an attitude toward the self. More generally, the term is used to describe a confidence in one's own value or abilities.*

and feel pleased or proud of their actions and choices. They can appreciate their uniqueness and accomplishments or be satisfied with a job well done.

Help your child understand that their feelings of self-worth will be a strong determining factor in who they choose to date and marry. A person who feels small and ashamed and thinks they are not good enough will often attract similar people.

## Start the Conversation

Explain that the foundation for a healthy sexuality comes from our feelings of self-worth. How we think of ourselves deeply affects how we interact with others. It also impacts our desires, decisions, and actions toward relationships, intimacy, and sex. These feelings of self-worth are often intertwined with our body image, our accomplishments, and our experiences while growing up. Talk about how good decisions and poor decisions impact our sense of self-worth.

Discuss ways people build their self-worth through positive self-talk, accomplishing goals, being kind to others, working hard, finding meaningful service, learning new things, etc. Ask your child what decisions they are most proud of and what they like most about their personality. What positive

# "Believe in yourself! Have faith in your abilities! Without a humble but reasonable confidence in your own powers you cannot be successful or happy."

-NORMAN VINCENT PEALE

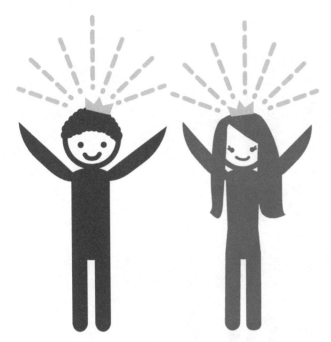

loves your child. It is because that person wants their own physical gratification.

Remind your child that under the right circumstances, sex can be positive and connecting. However, under the wrong circumstances, it can also be damaging and demeaning. Tell your child that they have a lot of power over how their sexual experiences will be. Using your personal values, discuss what the right circumstances and the wrong circumstances are for sex. Feel free to connect this discussion with lesson #3: "Emotional Intimacy."

outcomes do they contribute to their family, church, and school? Tell your child what you are most proud of in your life.

Ask your child to explain the following sentence. A person who respects themselves will not demean others. Is this true? Why or why not? How does this apply to friendships? How does this apply to romantic relationships?

Talk about how some people may engage in sexual activities as a way to boost their sense of self-worth. Explain that many people equate sex with love, thinking that if someone wants to have sex with them, that person must love them or want a relationship with them. Discuss the folly of this way of thinking. Teach your child that love is selfless, thoughtful, and not ruled by physical desire and lust. If a person is pushing your child for sex before they are fully committed, it is not because that person

## Questions for Your Child

Q True self-worth is never based on our looks, the clothes we wear, or what kind of house we live in. What things can you do and what decisions can you make to feel proud of yourself?

Q Are self-esteem and self-worth built by taking care of yourself emotionally and physically? Are they built by believing that you are worthy of respect and dignity simply for being a human being?

Q How does your self-worth affect your decisions with friends? With romantic relationships?

Q Often, a person's feelings of self-worth determine whether they will become sexually active or whether they will stay in certain relationships. What can you do to make sure your relationships are a reflection of valuing yourself?

- If you feel good about yourself, how might you treat someone else? If you feel bad about yourself, how might you treat someone else?
- How might a person who feels good about themselves approach sex differently from someone who does not?
- Is it better to be alone than to be with someone who pressures you?
- How do you know if you really want sex or if you're just going along with it?
- Should you act in the moment or make a decision about having sex ahead of time?
- How can you live without regrets?

## Activity

Gather your family or a group of your child's friends together. Give everyone a small note card and a pen. Have each person write their name on the top of the card, then pass the card to their left. When they receive a new note card, they should write something they admire or like about the person named on the card. Encourage the group to write deeper, more meaningful compliments than "nice" or "sweet." You may have the group share some of what was written or not. Tell them to put their note card in their wallet or a place where they will see it and review it often.

## Additional Resources:

"8 Things Your Daughter Needs to Hear from YOU" from Educate and Empower Kids
Written for mothers to their daughters, this article lists the top eight things that every daughter needs to hear.

"5 Ways a Mother Can Develop Self-Worth in Her Son" from Educate and Empower Kids
Written for mothers to their sons, this article lists five things that can be done to help improve self-worth.

"5 Things a Father Can Do to Increase His Daughter's Self-Worth" from Educate and Empower Kids
Written for fathers to their daughters, this article talks about five things that fathers can do for their daughters to improve their daughters' self-worth.

"Taking 'Hotness' Out of Your Kids' Self-Worth Equation" from Educate and Empower Kids
This wonderful article teaches about how children are worthy of love and so much more without worrying excessively about how they look.

# 14.
# Liking Yourself

With so much negativity surrounding our kids at school, on social media, and elsewhere, it is imperative for them to have a consistent place and people who care for them and can remind them of just how special and wonderful they are. We can help our children see the amazing talents, interests, and characteristics that make them unique.

Take time to discuss some of the distractions, situations, challenges, or even people that might cause your child to dislike themself or doubt themself and the talents they have.

Express your love and confidence in your child. Let them know that they are entitled to deep relationships and genuine intimacy and that they are capable of making great decisions. Acknowledge and remind your child what's remarkable about them. Each day, make some small effort to remind your child that they are important and that you know they are capable of exceptional things.

## Start the Conversation

It's important that your child recognizes and acknowledges what's great about them. Everyone has special talents, interests, mannerisms, and characteristics that make them the unique person they are. Appreciating what's great about yourself is the basis of liking yourself. When you like yourself, you know that you're entitled to great relationships and genuine intimacy. You are also more confident in your ability to make great decisions. Having a strong foundation of liking oneself will pave the way to future successes.

 **POSITIVE SELF-TALK:** *Anything said to oneself for encouragement or motivation, such as phrases or mantras; also, one's ongoing internal conversation with oneself, like a running commentary, which influences how one feels and behaves.*

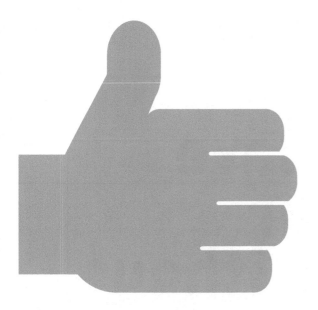

Help your child celebrate who they are and encourage the special qualities you see in them by talking about your impression of them. Give specific examples of things they've done or said that you admire or thought were impressive. Sometimes it's hard for a kid to see the good in themself, so point out to them what they've done well: tell your child five to 50 things that are awesome about them. You can even continue to do this throughout their lives. In this way you can be a mirror for them to help show them the fantastic people they are!

Teach them what positive self-talk is. Teach them how critical it can be to speak kindly to ourselves if we are to survive in a harsh world where there is so much negativity around us. Emphasize to your teenager that no one expects them to be perfect; we all make mistakes, but they are destined for greatness.

Discuss self-worth: what it is, where it comes from, and how it affects relationships. Please see the glossary for more information. Let your teen know that what they do or don't do sexually is not the sum total of who they are. Talk to your teen about the option of waiting to have sex. Explain that one usually can't have great sex without knowing how to have great intimacy. But also remind your child that if they have been sexually active and regret it, it should not overshadow their self-worth or define who they are. Reinforce that they are still learning and will continue to grow in their capability to make healthy decisions for themselves.

## Questions for Your Child

Q What do you like about yourself? In your journal, write down a list of at least 5 things that make you unique!

Q What are some of your strengths?

Q What are some circumstances that make it difficult to think well of yourself?

Q How is sex linked with liking yourself?

Q Do you think differently of friends who have had sex versus friends who have not?

Q Will you think more or less about yourself after becoming sexually active? Or will you feel the same about yourself?

Q What are the healthy emotional and intellectual elements a person should have before having sex? Do you have all of those healthy elements?

"Believe in yourself! Have faith in your abilities! Without a humble but reasonable confidence in your own powers you cannot be successful or happy."

-NORMAN VINCENT PEALE

## Activity

Ask your child to write down a recent time when they used negative self-talk internally. Then, ask the following questions:

- Q What were the circumstances of that situation?
- Q Would you talk to other people like you talk to yourself?
- Q Why is negative self-talk futile and sometimes destructive?
- Q What do you think would happen if you started talking more kindly to yourself?

### Sample Scenario

Pose the following scenario to your teen to give this subject a real-life context:

There's a popular group of kids at school that is known for having parties involving alcohol and casual sex. Part of you is secretly a little in awe of them and sometimes you imagine being a part of the group. Now you've been invited to one of these parties.

- Q How will you decide what to do?
- Q What questions could you ask yourself to discover what draws you to this group?
- Q How will you feel about yourself if you go?
- Q How will you feel about yourself if you drink and possibly have sex under those circumstances?

## Additional Resources:

"Lesson: Learning Positive Self-Talk" from Educate and Empower Kids
In this family lesson, parents have the opportunity to teach and practice using positive self-talk with their children.

"Empower Your Child Today Through Positive Self-Talk and Affirmations" from Educate and Empower Kids
This amazing article explains the importance of positive self-talk and provides examples of affirmations that parents and children can use.

"Self-Harm: A Major Concern for Parents in the Digital Age" from Educate and Empower Kids
This article talks from a parent's personal experience with a child. It expounds on how to recognize self-harm and what the best methods of dealing with it are.

# 15.
# Body Image & Sex

Body image involves more than just how your teen thinks their body looks; it also involves how those beliefs impact your teen's thoughts and feelings about themselves. Body image includes the desire to be attractive to others. It's entwined with one's self-worth. Countless people mentally beat themselves up because they loathe their appearance.

A poor body image impacts relationships with others and can also affect one's sex life. Someone with a negative body image may not want to be naked with another person or may avoid sex because of how their body looks.

Body image is also not just a "girls issue." Many boys struggle with their body image. You may find "A Lesson About Healthy Body Image" and "Lesson: Teaching Healthy Body Image to Boys" useful in these discussions.

If possible, discuss with your spouse or other supporting figure what you can do to help a child who is struggling with a negative body image. Think critically about how your words and actions have impacted your kids' body image. Have you always been positive about your looks in front of your children?

Body image is an important topic that warrants in-depth discussion. You can find further resources on educateempowerkids.org. Though geared toward younger children, you will also find the workbooks of *Messages About Me: Sydney's Story, A Girl's Journey to Healthy Body Image* and *Messages About Me: Wade's Story, A Boy's Quest for Healthy Body Image* especially helpful in body image discussions with people of all ages.

 **BODY IMAGE:**
*An individual's feelings regarding their own physical appearance, attractiveness, and/or sexuality. These feelings and opinions are often influenced by other people and media sources.*

## Start the Conversation

Explain that developing a healthy body image can improve a person's feelings of self-worth. How your teenager feels about their body affects how they feel about themself, which is a key indicator of what kind of relationships/friendships they make. Share your feelings about your body and struggles you may have had with your own body image.

Acknowledge to your child that there's a lot of pressure on teenagers in regard to their appearance. Discuss the many amazing things everyone's body can do, like healing itself and allowing us to see, hear, taste, feel, learn, run, cry, dance, laugh, and generally experience the world. If your child can learn to appreciate these things, they are much more likely to develop a healthy body image. Ask your teen to name at least 10 things their body can do. If your teen feels like they want to improve their health and appearance, talk about healthy eating, exercising, sleeping, and drinking of water. Explain that fad diets do not have long-lasting effects and can be generally unhealthy.

Our culture is enormously focused on appearance. Even though we know that a person's character and "inner beauty" are more important, we are influenced by the media's obsession with looks. Discuss media influences and how narrow ideas of beauty affect all people. Discuss how edited digital images and films show impossible standards (more on this in the next lesson, #16, "Being Media Savvy").

## Questions for Your Child

Q How does body image affect our inherent sense of value?

Q Why is it sometimes so difficult to like our appearance? Is it because of unattainable media images? Have we learned to dislike our looks from family members or friends?

Q How can you prevent others' opinions from influencing what you think about yourself?

Q What do you like best about the way you look? Is there anything you'd like to change?

Q Do you have friends who are critical of their bodies? What can you say to help them appreciate all that their bodies can do?

Q How can we replace the negative self-talk about our behaviors or bodies that sometimes come into our minds?

Q Would you date someone you like but don't think is attractive?

Q Besides looks, what are some other things that attract us to people?

Q How would your body image affect your ability to enjoy sex?

Q Why do you think some people avoid sex if they think they are too fat or too thin, or if they have other reservations about the way they look?

## Activity

Thoroughly discuss each of the following points. Take time to think and see where you can incorporate these ideas into your daily life. (From "More Than a Body," YA Weekly, August 2019).

1. **"See your body as an instrument, not an ornament.** Think of your body as a tool for experiencing life, not just something to be looked at. Focus on how you feel and what you can do.

2. **Try a media cleanse or fast.** Try taking a break from media [especially social media] and then take inventory of what you're viewing when you go back. Do the images you see or the accounts you follow spark anxiety or shame? Do they objectify people? If so, you have the power to unfollow, unsubscribe, and fill your feed with goodness.

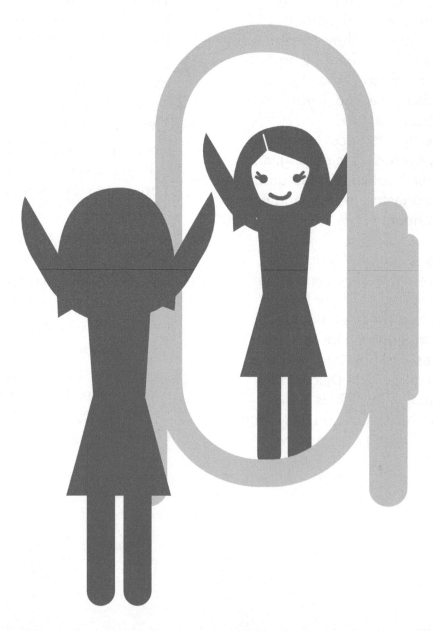

3. **Take responsibility for your own thoughts and actions.** Regardless of what anyone else wears or does, you can decide to view them as a person, not an object. Respect others' agency to make choices that are different from yours and treat them with dignity.

4. **Join forces with others to see more and be more.** Ask friends and family to join you in rejecting objectifying media and conversation. Speak up about the importance of seeing ourselves and others as more than a body, and back it up by how you talk about yourself and others."

> Teaching your kids about body gratitude and praising them wisely are two critical steps you can take as a parent to help your kids love their bodies for exactly what they are—
> which is a living, breathing, beautiful miracle.

## Additional Resources:

"Teaching Our Kids Body Gratitude: A Critical Skill in Our Image-saturated World" from Educate and Empower Kids
This article offers detailed suggestions for how parents can help teach their children about body positivity and how they can help boost their children up.

"Building a Better Body Image: 4 Ways to Boost Yours and Your Kids' Self-Worth" from Educate and Empower Kids
This article goes through different problems that many people have with self-esteem and includes tips on how to counter those, for both parents and kids.

"Inspiring Positive Body Image in Kids in a Social Media Age" from About Progress
This podcast episode discusses how parents can encourage positive body image at home.

"Helping a Child Who is Overweight Have a Positive Body Image" from Educate and Empower Kids
Similar to the above link, this article goes through a few strategies on how to increase a healthy body image in children who are already struggling with it.

# 16.
# Being Media Savvy

Media is a powerful tool for those doing good, but also for the nefarious. Many websites, books, magazines, TV shows, movies, and songs contain compelling sexual content that tries to convince us that a person's sexiness is one of their most, if not the most, important attributes.

In generations past, it was essential to understand how to truly comprehend the written word. Now, it is also important to be able to deconstruct the many pictures and video messages in our image-based culture. Encourage your child to think critically about the images they see and the messages that are being relayed. Help them see how images and words are manipulated in order to promote a particular reaction or interpretation.

Check out our free ebook A Family's Guide to Digital Media on our website—a super helpful resource in finding a media balance for your family by providing you the tools to create your own family media usage plan.

## MEDIA LITERACY:
*The ability to study, understand, and sometimes create messages in various media such as movies, social media posts, games, music, news stories, online ads, etc. It also includes understanding how to navigate being online, what to avoid, and what information to share and/or keep private.*

## Start the Conversation
Consider with your child how many hours a week you as a family are spending on media. Teach your teen to deconstruct images by understanding who the audience for the media images is, what the images are trying to communicate or sell, and why those particular people were used for the images. Teach your teenager that advertisers have a vested interest in us feeling bad about ourselves and therefore buying their products and "miracle" remedies.

ASK YOURSELF THIS QUESTION:

# Who do you want telling your child what they should look like and who they should be?

Teach your child the concept of media literacy, including critical thinking and dissecting an image and the subtle messages in advertisements. The more you do, the more educated and empowered this generation of consumers will be.

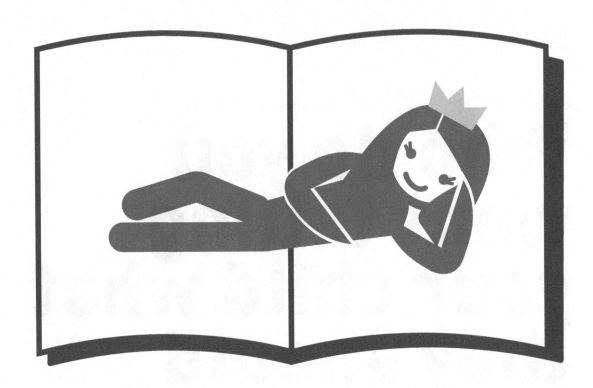

Explain to your child that many media images and messages are trying to sell something and do not represent a true reality. Advertisers and others often use sex because it's a powerful tool in grabbing people's attention.

Point out that people come in all shapes and sizes because we're not meant to all be the same, but the media usually only portrays a narrow vision of beauty. Emphasize that the people in media images have frequently been digitally touched up or Photoshopped.

## Questions for Your Child

- Q How does the media portray beauty?
- Q How does the media portray sexual relationships?

- Q How can you be true to yourself in a culture of powerful media messages?
- Q Does the media reflect the general attitudes about sex and relationships you see in your daily life?
- Q Are your personal values and attitudes reflected in popular books, movies, or TV shows?
- Q What do you think about the relationships and behaviors you see in the media?
- Q How can you create your own ideas about sex and relationships separate from a culture of powerful media messages?
- Q How many hours a week are we as a family spending on media? Are we unplugging enough to have meaningful relationships with each other?

## Activity

Teach your child to deconstruct images—a skill that everyone should practice, not just kids! Together, look at an ad in a magazine, online, or anywhere. Practice breaking it down to see the real message by discussing the questions provided. This same activity can be done with movies, music, news, and even social media feeds!

### Ask the following questions:

○ What is the overall message? Why was this ad made?

○ What did they use to sell this product? (Objects, words, font styles, Photoshop, etc.)

○ How does this advertisement make you feel? What do the creators want us to do?

○ What are some of the underlying or hidden messages?

○ What values were emphasized? What values were excluded?

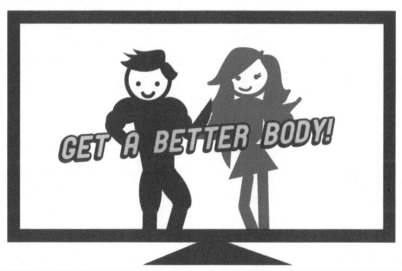

## Additional Resources:

"Media Literacy II: Teaching Kids How to Deconstruct Images" from Educate and Empower Kids
In this family lesson, teach your kids to deconstruct media messages, so they can avoid the pitfalls of low self-worth when comparing themselves to false advertising and social media messages.

"Creating a Media Guideline for Your Family" from Educate and Empower Kids
"A media guideline is a great tool for protecting your family from online dangers and excessive usage of devices."

"Media Literacy: Ads Sell More Than Products to Our Kids" from Educate and Empower Kids
This article talks about the different techniques ads tend to use to sell products and also manipulate how consumers feel about themselves and said products. It then talks about how to help your child not fall for the tricks of advertising.

# 17.
# Pornography

Our children are being exposed to pornography at a very young age, and because of that, many are forming increasingly unhealthy attitudes about sex, love, and intimacy. Porn has become a huge influence as it trickles into and hypersexualizes all aspects of popular culture, including television, advertising, toys, games, language, and dating.

Unsurprisingly, the use of porn is linked with increased callousness toward sex, decreased satisfaction with the user's sexual partner, acceptance of the rape myth (that women like it and want to be raped), and disconnect from real-life relationships.

Most of our teenagers have already been exposed to porn, so it's important for us to approach this topic calmly and rationally. Don't freak out! Rather, be frank with your child and ask them frank questions.

For more detailed help, check out our book *How to Talk to Your Kids About Pornography* and our website www. educateempowerkids.org for timely family lessons and more.

## Start the Conversation

First, make sure you and your teen are on the same page by asking them what they think pornography (porn) is. Ask them when the first time they saw it was. Then, ask when the last time was. If they seem embarrassed, reassure your child that it's normal to be curious and that you love them no matter what.

**PORNOGRAPHY:**
*The portrayal of explicit sexual content for the purpose of causing sexual arousal. In it, sex and bodies are commodified for the purpose of making a financial profit. It can be created in a variety of media contexts, including videos, photos, animation, books, and magazines. Its most lucrative means of distribution is through the internet.*

Next, explain how porn can damage individuals. Just as with drugs and alcohol, teenage brains are ill-equipped to deal with porn. Extended pornography use affects the brain chemistry and can lead to addictive behaviors (see glossary), decreased empathy, dissatisfaction, and a diminished view of women. For more information, check out one of our online articles, "8 Harmful Effects of Pornography on Individuals."

Explain that mixed reactions and feelings—being simultaneously repulsed, excited, disgusted, and aroused—are normal because of intense chemical reactions in the brain and body when viewing porn. Talk about how the flood of intense pleasure chemicals can lead to addiction. If you feel it's appropriate, share with your child any experience you've had with pornography and how it made you feel.

Discuss how porn use damages relationships. Pornography can cause problems with trust and desensitize users to their partner's humanity and individuality. It puts the focus on the user's own pleasure and satisfaction without regard to their partner's. It's also important to note that the growing rate of erectile dysfunction in the male population is linked to prolonged exposure to and use of pornography.

Talk about how pornography is damaging our society. The millions of people viewing porn has promoted the spread of rape culture (see glossary), especially when most pornography features women in positions of inferiority and powerlessness. It leads to a collective loss of empathy and to the idea that women should always be sexually available. The proliferation of porn has led to a hypersexualized culture where even food, pets, and children are sexualized.

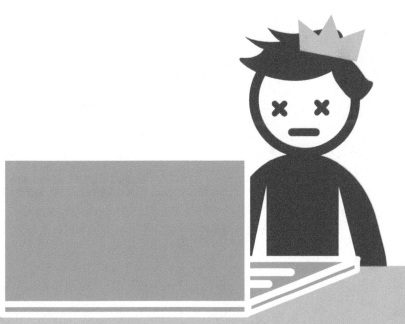

# "No parent can child-proof the world. A parent's job is to world-proof the child."

-DOUG FLANDERS

## Questions for Your Child

- Why doesn't porn depict warm, loving, intimate relationships?

- Why does the violence in porn seem to "disappear" when it is combined with sex? Why do some people accept that a woman must "want it" or "like it" (slapping, name-calling) if sex is involved?

- If you are having a tough day or are bored and want to see something online that you know you shouldn't, what are some other activities you can do to distract yourself? (Read, talk with a friend, take a nap, play a board game, ride a bike, etc.)

- Besides what was mentioned in the lesson, how else is pornography damaging to individuals AND relationships? How is it damaging to society?

- Have you ever been in a situation where you were shown something pornographic and you felt uncomfortable? How did you handle it?

- How do your friends feel about porn?

- Where are we most likely to encounter porn? At home? At school?

- How could using porn affect your view of other people?

- What are the crucial elements of healthy sex that porn destroys?

- Some people seek out porn when bored, lonely, tired, sad, or stressed out. What do you do when you have these types of feelings? How do you cope?

## Additional Resources:

"Signs and Symptoms of Porn Addiction in Kids" from Educate and Empower Kids
Here is a helpful article which lists some of the signs that your child might be struggling with pornography.

"A Lesson About Pornography—For Ages 12+" from Educate and Empower Kids
This is a great family lesson to further teach children about the dangers of online pornography and how to best prevent and combat it.

"Why Anti-Porn Is Not Equal to Anti-Sex" from Educate and Empower Kids
This article goes through the different reasons why being against porn doesn't mean being against sex.

"How to Get Kids Off Anime and Other Sexualized Media" from Educate and Empower Kids
Here are 8 tips to help you and your partner tackle concerns about hyper-sexualized media your children may be exposing themselves to.

"Ten Reasons Why You Need to Talk to Your Child About Porn" from Educate and Empower Kids
It's a tough topic, we know, but this article explains many of the reasons it's so necessary to talk to kids about what porn is, how damaging it is, and how to avoid it.

# 18.
# Masturbation

Some parents consider this to be the most awkward of all sexual conversations they have with their kids. That's okay. You can do this! Just be real and be compassionate as you approach this topic.

Think about your definition of masturbation and what actions you think constitute masturbation. What are your thoughts on this topic? Do you think masturbation is healthy? Why or why not? Think about these questions and get comfortable! Be ready to talk about your views on masturbation and about the consequences of making masturbation a habit or a coping mechanism for stress, boredom, or loneliness.

Even though (medically) the behavior can be a normal part of a teen's development, there are other reasons parents may wish to discourage masturbation. Do you have personal or religious views that are different from the medical view that masturbation is healthy? Whatever your views, it is critical that you avoid any language or actions that imply that masturbation is shameful. Since masturbation often accompanies pornography viewing, you may wish to discuss this lesson in conjunction with lesson #17, "Pornography."

Most kids masturbate for the simple reason that it feels good. Occasionally, they may engage in compulsive masturbation because they have been sexually abused by an adult or peer. In this case, deeper resources and therapy may be necessary.

 **MASTURBATION:** *Self-stimulation of the genitals in order to feel sexual pleasure and/or orgasm.*

## Start the Conversation

First, discuss what masturbation is. Without using shame or negative language, discuss your family values and opinions on masturbation. Point out that many teenagers use masturbation as a coping mechanism or an escape. Ask your child what they think the consequences are of making it a habit. Discuss the pros and cons of forming various habits over their lifetime. Teens may also use pornography as a coping mechanism. Discuss a variety of healthy coping mechanisms: going for a run or working out, taking a few deep breaths, reading a book, playing a game, doing yoga, or talking to someone you love and trust.

Discuss the role puberty may play in becoming interested in masturbation, such as boys having spontaneous erections and both boys and girls being flooded with new hormones. Whether your teen masturbates or not, it is still important they understand their own body. This includes how it looks and what function EVERY body part plays. Consider encouraging your daughter to use a mirror to look thoroughly at her vulva, labia, and vagina.

## Questions for Your Child

Q  What constitutes masturbation?

Q  Do you feel that masturbation is healthy? Why or why not?

Q  Is it healthy to explore our bodies? Is there a difference between masturbating and exploring?

Q  How can exploring our bodies make us feel more comfortable with ourselves?

Q  What have you heard about using masturbation as a coping mechanism or an escape?

Q  Are there any consequences to making masturbation a habit? Do you think it can be a healthy habit or is it always wrong?

Q  Should masturbation replace a relationship?

Q  Why does it seem that our culture is more accepting of boys masturbating than girls?

## Additional Resources:

"Talking With Our Kids About Masturbation–Without Shame!" from Educate and Empower Kids
"Masturbation should not play a major role in your child's life, either as a source of relentless guilt or as a frequent and persistent habit that displaces healthy sexual relations in the future."

"Talking With Our Daughters About Masturbation" from Educate and Empower Kids
Masturbation is an important topic that needs to be addressed with both boys and girls. This article goes into how to do so, specifically with your daughters.

"Masturbation and Kids–Moving Beyond the Shame!" from Educate and Empower Kids
A personal story is shared about a girl's experience with masturbation and the shame that she felt. She tells how she recovered and worked through the feelings of shame.

# 19.
# Shame & Guilt

Everyone makes mistakes. We miscalculate, we misjudge, and we misconstrue. We fall down and then must pick ourselves back up. Thankfully, we learn and improve so that these mistakes can be for our good.

The point of this lesson is to help your child understand the difference between guilt and shame and how to appropriately deal with guilt and leave shame out of their lives. Consider reading the articles in the additional resources section before discussing this lesson with your child.

## Start the Conversation

First, remind your child that all of us are human and make mistakes. All of us are progressing through life in different ways, and every single day, we make mistakes. We must decide if we are going to let those mistakes define us or if we are going to try to be better.

Discuss the difference between guilt and shame. Guilt can be a healthy means of prompting us to make a change in our lives. Feelings of shame usually translate into negative feelings toward ourselves, and they focus on the thought, "I am a bad person." By contrast, guilt is usually easier to resolve and translates into "I made a mistake and I need to fix it." Talk about what steps could be taken to avoid and resolve feelings of shame.

Explain to your child that curiosity about sex is natural and nothing to feel guilt or shame over. Remind them that it is also natural to become aroused by different experiences and that there is no shame in that either. Talk about how sex was often not discussed at all in past generations. Then reflect on, and share some of the things your parents or teachers may have inadvertently (or purposely) taught you about sex in a shame-based way.

**GUILT:**
 is the feeling that you made a mistake that needs to be remedied.

**SHAME:**
is the feeling that your whole self is wrong or bad.

## Questions for Your Child

Q What are some experiences that we may feel shame over?

Q When we have made a mistake, how can we stop ourselves from feeling shame and instead focus on what we can do to make things better and move forward?

Q Who could you talk to if you have feelings of shame?

Q If you feel guilty about something, how can you remedy those feelings?

Q What will you do if you feel ashamed or guilty about something you've done or seen?

Q Why do some people think sex is "bad" or "dirty"?

Q What situations could cause guilt or shame about sex?

Q What are society's standards for sex? Does our family agree with society's standards?

Q Under what circumstances is sex a good, positive act?

Q Why is it natural to be curious about sex?

Q Is it okay for girls and boys to become aroused?

Q Sometimes kids and adults who have been sexually abused feel shame or blame themselves for what was done to them. Why do you think this happens? How can they reclaim a sense of healthy sexuality?

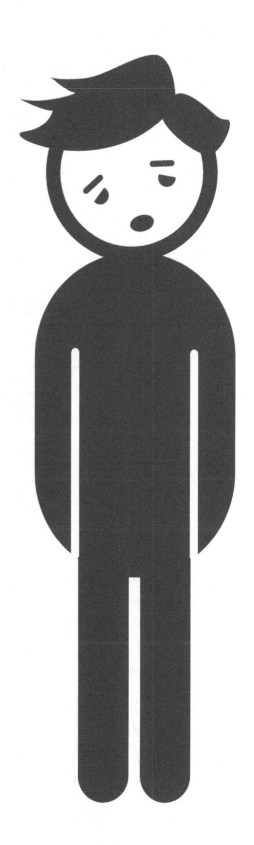

## Activity

Help your child really understand the difference between guilt and shame. Share an experience that you felt guilt over. Tell your child how you remedied your guilt. Now share a time where you felt shame. Explain what that felt like and how you were able to make peace with yourself. Ask others in your family to share an experience with either guilt or shame and how they overcame those feelings.

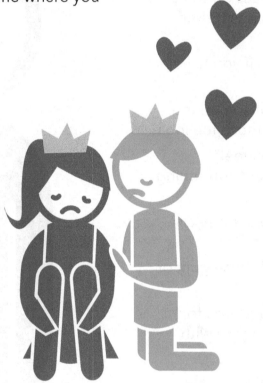

---

## Additional Resources:

"Three Mistakes I've Made Using Shame and Guilt" from Educate and Empower Kids
This article describes some of the ways we may inadvertently teach our children to associate shame and guilt with body image and behavior.

"Teaching Without Shame: Understanding Your Child's Curiosity" from Educate and Empower Kids
This article helps parents understand how to be calm and handle their children's curiosity without having them feel embarrassed.

"Stop the Mom Shame! Three Ways We Can Be Kinder to Ourselves" from Educate and Empower Kids
Shame can affect us all, especially moms who feel the pressure of raising kids in every way we feel they need to be, but this mentality negatively affects both us and our kids.

"For Survivors of Sexual Abuse: How to Talk to Kids About Healthy Sexuality" from Educate and Empower Kids
This article goes through a few different tactics a sexual abuse survivor could use when teaching healthy sexuality to kids, and talks about how much shame thrives in secrecy.

The best way we can strengthen our children against the mixed societal messages regarding sexuality, guilt, and shame is to **practice honesty,** even when it means correcting possible past mistakes.

# 20.
# Sexting & Social Media

Although social media is a handy tool for adults, it has been linked to increased anxiety, feelings of inadequacy, depression, and feelings associated with poor body image, especially among teenagers. This is in large part because many people use social media to compare their worst to others' curated, filtered images. Help your child avoid pain and suffering by

 **SEXTING:** *The sending or distribution of sexually explicit images, messages, or other material via phones, email, or instant messaging.*

WAITING to give them a smartphone for as long as possible (or don't give them a smartphone at all)! The use of "dumb" phones is on the rise again with great mental health benefits for kids. Sexting, or sharing nudes, has become very prevalent among adults AND teens. The legal ramifications of sexting are such that even an innocent receiver of a nude

picture can get in trouble for having it. It is considered child pornography if it depicts naked pictures of people under 18 years old, which is illegal to solicit, create, send, or store. The legal consequences for having or distributing it could fall under child pornography or child exploitation laws. A person who has been found with nude photos of teenagers may face jail time and/or be placed on the sex offender registry. Our book *Conversations With My Kids: 30 Essential Family Discussions for the Digital Age* and the lessons on our website can help you with these and many other vital family talks.

## Start the Conversation

Discuss with your child the explosion of social media use, which has also given rise to an upsurge of a free-for-all mentality. People frequently share opinions, thoughts, and comments unchecked. People can be blunt, rude, and callous in their use of social media. "Show, don't tell" your child how to be good digital citizens by being kind and respectful in your own social media interactions! Remind your child that EVERYTHING shared on social media can have an impact that we might never expect.

Consider doing the following to help your child interact online:

- Show your child how to handle a disagreement on social media.
- Show your child healthy and unhealthy examples of social media use.
- Discuss what to do if your child receives a nude photo via direct message or text.
- Teach them to be thoughtful online and in person.
- Encourage as much face-to-face interaction as possible with your child and their friends—including group dating—as a balance to their online socialization.

Don't forget to emphasize the importance and benefit of face-to-face communication! Explain how using primarily social media, texting, and other electronic communication to "interact" with others causes a disconnect between people and a sense of distance and removal that can lead to inappropriate behavior online.

Even if you think your child would never send a nude or explicit photo, please talk to them about it! Make sure you are on the same page by asking your child what they know about sexting and if they know of kids sending nude photos at their school. Create a plan for what your child should do if someone shows them nude photos or if they receive a sext or nude.

Talk about empathy and seeing a person for who they are and not just as body parts. Discuss the double standard when it comes to sharing nudes in our culture. People often do not shame a boy for requesting a nude photo of a girl, but they will shame a girl for sending one. Ask your child why this double standard might exist.

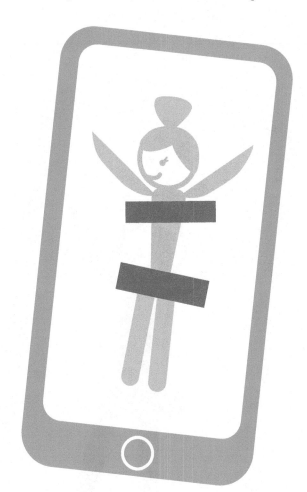

## Questions for Your Child

- Why do so many teens and adults spend hours each day on social media?
- Does the time you spend using various technologies increase or diminish your capacity to live, to love, and to serve in meaningful ways?

Q What might make people think they can say anything they want on social media, regardless of the effects? Why do people feel they can say things on social media that they would never say face-to-face?

Q What is appropriate use and behavior on social media? What behavior is not okay?

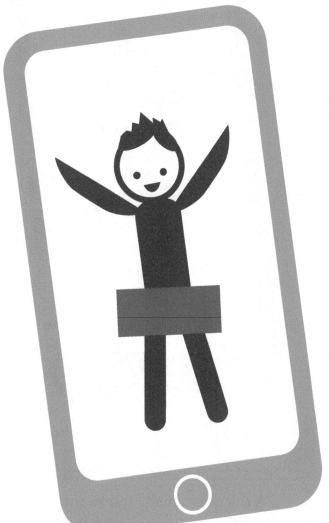

Q What are some ways we can help and uplift others with social media?

Q Are you the same person online that you are in real life?

Q How can you nurture real-life relationships?

Q What kind of face-to-face time is needed to maintain a healthy relationship? How will you balance your electronic communications with "the real thing"? What might it say about a person if they ask or demand nude photos of someone else? How do you think a person might feel when someone requests or demands a partially or fully nude photo of them?

Q What do your friends think of sexting? Have you or any of your friends been asked to send nudes? Have any of your friends asked for nude photos from a classmate?

Q Once you have sent a photo, can you ever get it back? Do you really think teens who ask for a nude photo will keep it to themselves?

Sexting is the act of sending sexual messages or pictures through a text or online. It has become a pervasive social norm among today's youth. It only takes one bad breakup or one jealous teenager for an image to go from being a private text to being an object of public consumption or ridicule.

## Additional Resources:

"6 Reason Why Kids Sext" from Educate and Empower Kids
This article goes through the various reasons why a teenager would sext, including things such as maturity and safety.

"Social Media and Teens: The Ultimate Guide to Keeping Kids Safe Online" from Educate and Empower Kids
This lesson walks you through how to set guidelines with your kids on social media in order to keep them safe from online dangers.

"Lesson: Talking to Your Kids About Sexting" from Educate and Empower Kids
"Chances are, your child will encounter this at some point in their life, either by unwittingly receiving a sext or feeling pressured to send one or actually sending one. This is why it's so important to talk to our kids about this growing and dangerous trend."

"Lesson: Uplifting Others Online and Everywhere" from Educate and Empower Kids
This family lesson helps kids to understand the importance of being kind both online and in person.

"Lesson: Teaching Our Kids Social Media Etiquette" from Educate and Empower Kids
"Teach your child the necessary manners associated with social media. Emphasize to them that as they practice and implement proper behaviors in their online lives, they will better understand the importance of using social media as a tool for good."

# 21.
# Sexual Conversations

Talking about sex can be fascinating, alluring, and even amusing—especially for teenagers. However, our kids need to know that they will often receive misinformation from other kids and pop culture, especially when it comes to the emotional and psychological aspects of sex. They also need to be taught that a peer or adult predator may use sexual conversations as a means of gauging how open or vulnerable your child may be to experimenting with sexual activity. Help your child understand who other appropriately suited adults are that they can talk about sex with.

As guardians, it is our duty to explain to and remind our teens that even if it is uncomfortable to approach the subject with us, we are still the best source of accurate information for them. Validate your child's feelings if they feel awkward talking about sex with you, but point out that you're empowering them with knowledge and that sex is good and healthy.

If your child asks you something that you don't know, be honest and tell them you will look it up and get back with them. And then make sure you follow up! Be sure you are discussing both the physical and emotional aspects of sexual topics.

> "A conversation is so much more than words: a conversation is eyes, smiles, and the silence between words." -ANNIKA THOR

## Start the Conversation

Let your teenager know that sex is a natural and important part of life that deserves time and discussion, but not with peers and certainly not with adults who are not 100% trustworthy (see activity below).

Tell your child: We as your parents (or guardians) will answer your questions and concerns with honest, reliable information. If there is something we don't know, we will find out together.

Discuss which people, beside yourself, you feel are appropriate to talk to about sex (a doctor at an appointment, a health teacher in a health class, a youth leader that you trust, etc.). Teach your child where they can find useful information about sex (anatomy books, etc.). Remind them that innocent internet searches for information about sex will usually take them to porn sites.

## Questions for Your Child

- Why is getting information about sex from other teenagers not the best choice?

- When it comes to us talking about sex together, are these conversations embarrasing, interesting, helpful, or something else?

- Do you think it's okay for an adult other than your parental guardians to discuss sex with you?

- Do you have any other trusted adults you could talk to about sex?

- Why is talking to people online about sex or other personal topics a terrible idea?

- Language and behavior is the expression of who we really are. What do your words and actions say about you? About what you think?

- In some social situations, boys and girls can say vulgar or rude comments with one another about sex or members of the opposite gender. Why might people do this?

- Many kids and teens think it's fun or cool to talk about sex in a crude or obscene way. Why is using clear and thoughtful words more effective in the long run?

- When it comes to sex, what are kids at school and your social circles talking about?

The words we choose
to speak or post online
have the power to build
others up or tear them
down. They can impact
the way others view us
and our interpersonal
relationships at school,
work, and home. When
we speak before thinking
or post something
inappropriate online,
it can have lasting
consequences on our
reputations and
affect the reputations
of others.

## Activity

### People We Trust

Can you remember any people in your youth that you thought were trustworthy or really cool, but you later realized were neither? Now imagine what it must be like for your child—dealing with people in person and online—trying to determine if those they interact with behind a screen are trustworthy or not. As much as we'd like to trust our children's judgment, their brains won't finish developing until at least age 22. This activity will show them what things to look for when judging someone's character and choosing which people to trust.

Get a piece of paper and pen and discuss which people in your community, family, or church you would trust with your children's lives. Ask your child to name two or three people they think are 100% trustworthy. Ask them about what makes them trustworthy. Share your views on what makes a person trustworthy. Be honest and blunt with your child. Explain why certain people do not make your list— this should be a very short list. If you have seen disturbing or troublesome behavior in certain people in your neighborhood or community, warn your child. But take care if you want to present troublesome behavior that is from one of their friends. They may become offended, start protecting this friend, and stop telling you things related to this person.

---

## Additional Resources:

"Lesson: Think Before You Speak, Post or Hit Send" from Educate and Empower Kids "Our words and posts create either positive or negative ripples, or small waves of change. They can influence others' perceptions, our own thinking, and the future course of our lives. Once we say something, it can be very hard to take it back; when we post something online, it is permanent."

"Lesson: Teaching Our Kids to Be Positive in Their Communication Online and In-Person" from Educate and Empower Kids This family lesson is intended to help kids learn to develop greater communication skills both in person and online.

"Is My Child Sexting? What Every Parent Needs to Know" from Educate and Empower Kids "Parents need to take a proactive role in teaching their children the appropriate use of technology and what their kids should do if they receive an inappropriate text or message."

"Teaching Our Kids: Your Online Actions Always Matter" from Educate and Empower Kids This article talks about how to teach your children that there are consequences to their actions in many forms than just what they can see. Understanding this is key in every interaction with others.

# 22.
# Sexual Identification

Our culture has become more open and quite accepting of different sexualities and lifestyles. Your child hears a lot more about it than you likely did at their age. It's important to discuss different aspects of sexual identification with your child.

Discuss various sexualities with respect and kindness. Many parents don't know for sure if their child is gay, straight,

**SEXUAL IDENTIFICATION:** *How one thinks of oneself in terms of whom one is romantically or sexually attracted to.*

transgender, or another sexuality. Be wise and compassionate as you approach this topic. See the glossary for definitions of straight/heterosexual, gay, lesbian, bisexual, transgender, non-binary, and intersex sexual identifications.

## Start the Conversation

Teach your teen that, although it influences all parts of their lives, sexuality is just one part of their lives. Their

sexuality is not the sum total of who they are. Our sexuality is an integral part of us as individuals, but it does not solely define us.

Take time to define and discuss what it means to be heterosexual (straight), homosexual (gay or lesbian), bisexual, transgender, queer, intersex, or non-binary. Ask your child to tell you about any other sexual identifications they have heard about. Explain that sexuality can be fluid, changing over time; it can also be constant. Ask your teen what factors might influence one's sexuality.

Explain that one's sexuality continues to develop and solidify during the teenage years. Tell your teen that their experiences should not be based on what they've seen in pornography, in sexualized media, or on social media. They have the right to understand and decide their own sexuality, have their own special experiences when the time is right, and formulate their own natural responses.

A great resource for understanding this further is available in our online article "Why We Need to Fight for Our Kids' Healthy Sexuality."

## Questions for Your Child

- ◯ What does LGBTQI stand for?
- ◯ What are your thoughts about different sexual identities?
- ◯ Are there kids in your school who are trans, gay, bi, etc.? How are they treated?
- ◯ Some say that sexuality can be fluid. What does that mean?
- ◯ How should everyone—LGBTQI or straight—be treated? How do you expect to be treated at school?
- ◯ How will you come to understand what your sexual identification is?
- ◯ What are the benefits of deciding for yourself what your sexual identity is (without reference to media such as porn or social media)?

- ◯ What roles come with being male or female? A member of society? A student in your school? A member of our family?

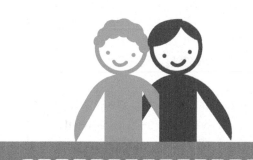

Having honest, open conversations with our children can also help to dispel any hateful or discriminatory statements that they may have heard or seen online that could be considered hurtful and inappropriate.

## Additional Resources:

"Starting Conversations With Your Kids About LGBTQ Identities" from Educate and Empower Kids
"It is important to teach through behavior and conversation that treating others with respect is critical to our communities. This will lead to more tolerance and safety for all people no matter their identity."

"How Teaching Healthy Sexuality Can Help Your Child Against the Predator, the Pressuring Partner, and the Prude" from Educate and Empower Kids
"Because the most important lesson about sexuality? Is that it is yours. It is personal and unique, and still healthy and normal."

"Understanding Gender Identity Terminology: A Guide for Parents" from Educate and Empower Kids
This article goes through the various different terms regarding LGBTQI and explains what each means.

"Guess Who's Coming to Dinner Now" from Educate and Empower Kids
This article goes through a few different ways to handle a coming-out situation with compassion and kindness.

# 23.
# Unwanted Sexual Attention

Women and girls used to deal with the majority of unwanted sexual attention, but now, more of our sons are facing sexual harassment from peers and adults. Help your child understand what unwanted sexual attention is. Emphasize that they can always say "no!"

Don't be afraid to be detailed and specific in referring to your child's options for getting out of an uncomfortable or dangerous situation. Let your child know that, even if they may have enjoyed certain attention before from a person, they still have the right to stop further attention at any time. Discuss how sexual attention can quickly escalate and how they need to trust their instincts. There is a reason why those alarm bells go off in their head or their stomach starts to churn.

Please remind your child that you are their biggest advocate and will help them in any situation you can! You may wish to combine this lesson with lesson #24, "How Predators Groom Kids."

## Start the Conversation

Begin by defining unwanted sexual attention—when a person gives any sexually based attention that your child does not want. This could be verbal or physical. Explain that it can come from anyone (friends, acquaintances, relatives, or strangers) or from anywhere (school, work, church, etc.). Regardless of the source, giving unwanted sexual attention is not okay!

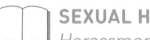 **SEXUAL HARASSMENT:** *Harassment involving unwanted sexual advances or obscene remarks. Sexual harassment can be a form of sexual coercion as well as an undesired sexual proposition, including the promise of reward in exchange for sexual favors.*

Talk about strategies for your teen to be aware of their surroundings and the people around them when they're in public places. Emphasize that there is no circumstance in which it is okay for someone to give them sexual attention that they don't want. Remind your child

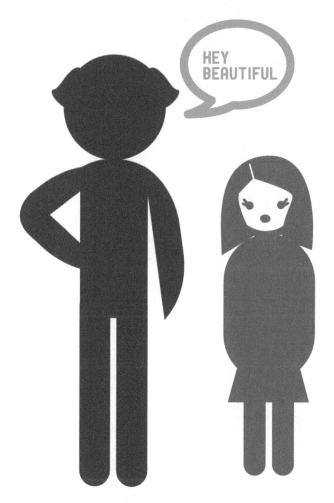

HEY BEAUTIFUL

that most cases of unwanted sexual attention and abuse come from people we know, not from strangers. Discuss safe places and people your child can go to if they are in an uncomfortable or dangerous situation.

Explain that there are many sexual behaviors that are illegal. Some include exposing genitals in public, harrasing someone with threats or sexual imagery via text or email, child sexual abuse material, an adult having sex with a minor, and rape. Refer to the information covered in lesson #10, "Consent."

## Questions for Your Child

- Q What are some examples of unwanted sexual attention? (Saying sexual things, asking for nude photos, touching someone's body without permission, etc.)

- Q What is sexual harassment? When might it happen to adults? To kids?

- Q What's the difference between a flirtatious compliment and unwanted sexual attention?

- Q Who should you talk to if someone is giving you unwanted sexual attention at school? At work?

- Q How could you help a friend, classmate, or teammate who is being sexually harassed?

- Q Why might a person give another person attention that's clearly not wanted?

- Q If someone gives you unwanted sexual attention (physical or verbal), are you at fault?

- Q Is it okay to tell the person giving unwanted attention to stop, even if it's a teacher, a coach, a church leader, or a relative? (YES!) Is it okay to defend yourself physically in order to get the person to stop?

Our kids can navigate the web with great deftness, but they lack the maturity and discernment needed to avoid dangers. It is precisely this combination of online prowess and immaturity that online predators are counting on to deceive children and teens and put them in harm's way. This is why it is imperative to teach them responsible behaviors, monitor their online use, and foster healthy open communication.

- How does pornography and our hypersexualized culture factor into people's ideas about sexual attention?
- If someone gives you unwanted sexual attention (physical or verbal) is this your fault?

## Activity

### What Will You Do?

Having a plan or knowing what to say in uncomfortable situations can be very empowering. Discuss the following and come up with a plan of how to deal with each scenario:

- A stranger whistles at you while you are walking down the street.
- A teacher rubs your shoulders, then does it again on another occasion.
- Your girlfriend/boyfriend asks you to send them a photo of you in your underwear.
- A classmate pinches you on your bottom.
- Your uncle begins tickling you and you feel uncomfortable.

*Feel free to add your own scenario! Ask your child if they have any scenarios they'd like to discuss.

## Additional Resources:

"What Online Predators Don't Want YOU to Do" from Educate and Empower Kids
This article discusses just how likely it is for children to encounter a predator, how it can happen, and what parents can do to protect their children.

"How to Identify A Child Predator Online" from Educate and Empower Kids
This article defines the various acronyms and terms used online that identify and describe sexual identifications, including those used by pedophiles.

"Peer on Peer Abuse: Why It Happens and What Parents Can Do" from Educate and Empower Kids
In this video, we talk about peer-on-peer abuse and what we as parents can do to prevent it.

# 24.
# How Predators Groom Kids

Most people are good, but there are predators in every culture, religion, and population. Predators can't be identified by how they look, where they live, or what their occupation is. They can be an uncle, a family friend, a neighbor, a stranger—anyone. They can be found online, at school, at church, and within our families. Be aware and make your child aware of what the warning signs and dangers of predators are and how predators groom their victims.

 **SEXUAL HARASSMENT:** *Someone who seeks to obtain sexual contact/ pleasure from another through predatory and/or abusive behavior. The term is often used to describe the deceptive and coercive methods used by people who commit sex crimes with a victim.*

Always listen to your children. Make it clear that you will not brush off their concerns if they ever feel not quite right about a person in their lives, no matter who it is. If your child reveals an incident of molestation or rape, take it seriously. Report it immediately.

Check out our helpful article "8 Ways a Predator Might Groom Your Child" and discuss common grooming behaviors with your teen.

## Start the Conversation

First talk about what a predator is and where they can be found (everywhere). Inform your child that 90% of sexual abuse is perpetrated by people we know, not strangers. Explain that most people are good and kind, but that we need to be aware that there are bad people in the world. These bad people can be anywhere in our communities and families. Use the previous lesson to discuss what counts as unwanted sexual attention, how your teen can get out of distressing or dangerous situations, and who they can turn to if something happens to them.

Predators are not just adults, even teenagers can learn to groom and prey on peers. Because of the huge increase in porn consumption by kids, there has

**Predators are generally our friends and family members in our community. They look just like us and know exactly how to hide in plain sight.**

been a considerable uptick in peer-on-peer abuse and assault. Talk about what it means to groom a person for sexual abuse or molestation. Grooming is essentially a predator incorporating themself into the teen's life through special attention, "test touching," and the gradual eroding of normal social boundaries in order to sexually abuse or molest the teen.

## A predator may use several methods to groom your child:

- Use "innocent," "affectionate" touching to desensitize and build trust
- Use their position of authority to manipulate
- Manipulate your child's need for love, attention, and affection
- Pay special attention to your child and make him feel important
- Touch your child in your presence to get you comfortable with their "affection"
- Work to become a close friend of the family
- Take advantage of natural curiosity about sex by telling dirty jokes, showing porn, or playing sexual games
- Present themself as a sympathetic listener when others disappoint your child

We have instincts that guide us and tell us when something doesn't feel right. Encourage your child to understand and identify their instincts and trust them. Even though instinctual feelings aren't perfect, following our instincts can help keep us safe.

## Questions for Your Child

Q Predators are not just adults, they can be other teenagers too. But teenage predators still use many of the same grooming techniques. What ways do predators groom their victims?

Q Predators have moved much of their activity online because this is where many kids and teens are "hanging out." Why is it important to keep your social media accounts private (and not public) and only accept friend requests from people you know?

Q People often feel embarrassed or ashamed to tell someone that they have been hurt or abused by a peer or adult. How can I, as your parent, help you to understand that I will always be on your side, believe you, and help you?

Q Why can it be difficult to stand up to adults? Would it be less difficult or more difficult to stand up to a peer or older teen?

Q How will you speak up when you don't feel quite right about someone? What if that someone is a family friend?

- Predators will usually single out a child/teen and try to spend time alone with them. What can you do to avoid being alone with a coach, teacher, or anyone that makes you feel uncomfortable?

- What could you do if you fear someone you know is being groomed?

## Sample Scenario

Pose the following scenario to your teen:

You're on the team and excited to be coached by Mr. M., a highly regarded coach. Several older friends have been coached by him, and their game improved significantly. You're hoping for the same improvement.

You're flattered when Coach M. starts paying special attention to you and your techniques. He begins touching you more, helping to correct your form. You start to feel a little uncomfortable about all the touching—it's kind of weird. Soon, Coach M. suggests setting up time after practice for the two of you to work together one-on-one. You feel very uncomfortable, even alarmed, at that idea.

### Ask the following questions:

- What will you do? Will you talk with someone you trust about your feelings?

- Will you suggest that a couple teammates join you?

## Additional Resources:

"The Secret I Almost Did Not Tell" from Educate and Empower Kids
The author tells of her personal experience with abuse and how she learned to teach her own children what to look for and what to avoid to protect themselves in the future.

"Child Predators: What Every Parent Should Know" from Educate and Empower Kids
This shows an Instructional video to help parents identify and protect children from predators.

"Protecting Special Needs Children From Unwanted Sexual Attention" from Educate and Empower Kids
This article goes through a few more ways to help educate and protect your child with special needs from people who would take advantage.

"Simple Ways to Protect Your Child From Common Abuse in the Digital Age" from Educate and Empower Kids
Here are some more examples of how predators may find access to your children, what to look out for, and how to prevent such contact.

"Sex Talks and Sexual Assault..." from Educate and Empower Kids
Though we wish no children would ever go through it, sexual assault happens frequently. If this has happened to your child, here is a compassionate and gentle approach to having those crucial sex talks with them.

# 25.
# Monogamy VS. Multiple Partners

In years past, discussing certain aspects of sexual health in a book for parents and families would have been unthinkable. However, with the increasing known variety of sexual activities and wider acceptance of such, it's become necessary for parents to educate themselves and their children on as many aspects of sexual health as possible.

As our culture embraces a larger variety of sexual behaviors, it seems that experts and nonexperts alike are unwilling to endorse any kind of limit on sexual health. When it comes to diet, exercise, medications, mental health practices, alcohol consumption, and sleep, there are specific guidelines and recommendations for how much is necessary and healthy and how much is too much. But when it comes to sex, few experts address the healthy or unhealthy limits of dating, sexual partners, prostitution, fetishes, etc.

For this reason, it is imperative that you think about and decide what limits and values you embrace and what you want your child to understand about the complexities of sexual relationships. Do you believe in monogamous relationships? If so, explain why.

If you feel that having multiple partners is healthy, clarify why.

Pop culture often portrays monogamous sex within marriage as confining. Do you agree with this? If so, explain why to your child. Talk about your views of casual sex and polyamory. Do you think it can be fulfilling and enjoyable, or lonely and empty? Share your thoughts.

Whatever lifestyle your child chooses to embrace, it's important for them to understand the freedom and peace of mind one has when they are true to themselves.

**MONOGAMY:** *Someone who seeks a relationship in which a person has one partner at any one time.*

**POLYAMORY:** *The practice of engaging in multiple romantic (and typically sexual) relationships, with the agreement of all the people involved.*

## Start the Conversation

Take time to discuss your family's standards and rules when it comes to becoming sexually active. Decide beforehand how you want to handle your child's possible questions about your own sexual history. Explain to your child how you feel about monogamy and the possible emotional and physical consequences to having casual sexual partners. Be prepared to handle and discuss anything your child may want to reveal to you about their own experiences.

Explain what polyamory is. Be honest, and clarify the possible emotional and spiritual benefits and disadvantages that having multiple partners can have on a person (particularly on women). Remind your child of the possible health risks of having multiple sexual partners; the possibility of contracting sexually transmitted diseases or infections (lesson #29) rises with each new sexual partner. See the glossary for definitions of STDs and STIs.

Share your wisdom and experience. Discuss when a person is mature enough to become sexually active. Should a person experiment with various partners of various genders? Express your views! You don't have to go into explicit details of your sexual experiences, but be willing to share your knowledge and understanding with your teen.

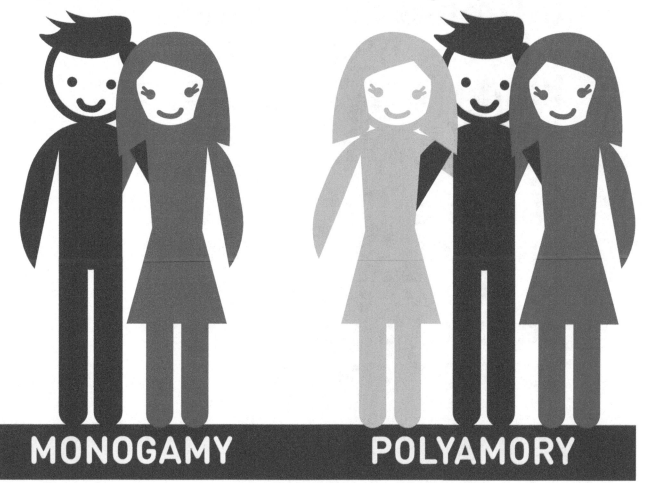

MONOGAMY          POLYAMORY

"Choosing a long-term or life-long partner (or partners) is among the most important decisions of your life. Whether you choose to be monogamous or polyamorous, your intimate relationship(s) will require courage, kindness, love, respect, and trust. So much of your future happiness can depend on your partner(s), so take time to get to know them before committing. You're worth it!"

-FRANKLIN VEAUX

## Questions for Your Child

- What do you think of monogamy? How do your friends feel about monogamy?

- How would monogamy impact your emotional health and physical health? How would having multiple sexual partners impact your emotional and physical health?

- Choosing a spouse is one of the most important decisions of your life. What will you use to guide you in choosing a partner for the rest of your life?

- Polyamory, or the practice of engaging in multiple romantic (and typically sexual) relationships, has become increasingly popular. Why do you think this is?

- Does our culture have different beliefs regarding men who have multiple partners versus women who have multiple partners? Why is that?

- Is the practice of having multiple sex partners at one time damaging to one's physical and mental health?

- Are there benefits to polyamoric relationships?

- Is it wise and ethical to have multiple partners at once without those partners knowing that's happening?

## Additional Resources:

"15 Things I Want My Son to Know About Love and Sex" from Educate and Empower Kids
This article offers a mother's perspective on what critical information she wants her own son to know about love and sex.

"15 Things I Want My Daughter to Know About Love and Sex" from Educate and Empower Kids
A mother's perspective on the best information her daughter should know about love and sex.

"For Parents: How to Have a Family Council" from Educate and Empower Kids
This family lesson helps you learn how to create a situation where you will be able to have these important conversations with your children.

# 26.
# Sex in a Committed Relationship VS Hook-Up Sex

In recent years the prevalence and acceptability of hook-up sex has increased dramatically. Emotionally, hookups can be tough for both men and women. Often one person in a hookup will expect different things than the other person and will leave the experience disappointed or worse. In addition, many people may engage in these behaviors because they think it's what they can get or because they feel that it's expecting too much to ask the other person to put in the effort of a committed relationship.

This discussion is meant to help your teen understand that sex is potentially one of the most vulnerable and special experiences they will ever have. They give certain emotional parts of themselves to friends, school, work, and family. But sex (the giving of both their body and their heart) is usually more fulfilling when given to just one person they deeply care about. Because of this, it is critical that they choose the right person to give their heart to.

However, you may guide this discussion in any way you choose, based on your experiences, wisdom, and values. If you think that sex is better in a committed relationship, clarify your reasons why. If you believe that hook-up sex is a fun, carefree alternative, explain why.

We can prepare our kids for their future sex lives with open, honest discussions. We must teach our kids the best we can so that when they do become sexually active, they will be able to judge for themselves whether it meets their personal needs or not.

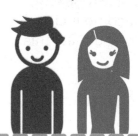

 **HOOK-UP SEX:** *A form of casual sex in which sexual activity takes place outside the context of a committed relationship. The sex may be a one-time event, or an ongoing arrangement. In either case, the focus is generally on the physical enjoyment of sexual activity without an emotional involvement or commitment.*

## Start the Conversation

Discuss your family's standards and expectations about sex within and outside of a committed relationship. Explain that hook-up sex is often promoted in pop culture as fun, easy, victimless, and without regrets. If you agree with this view, share your reasons. Feel free to talk about the realities of these pop culture ideas and how a person's feelings of self-worth will often help determine if a person will engage in hook-up sex or not.

Describe the traditional view that sex is better, more intimate, and more meaningful when in a committed relationship. Explain your personal views whether you agree or disagree.

Discuss how increased anxiety, shame, regret, a boosted ego, stereotyping, etc., can be associated with hookups. Take a few minutes to share with your child your thoughts and opinions about mobile apps, such as Kasual, Tinder, and Grindr, that promote hookups between local strangers.

## Questions for Your Child

- How is sex in a committed relationship different from casual hookups? Why might people have hook-up sex?

- What are the emotional aspects of sex in a committed relationship? Is there an emotional aspect to hookups?

- Why do you think people have hook-up sex?

- What emotional baggage might you be able to avoid by waiting to have sex until you are in a committed relationship? What are some other benefits of waiting to have sex until you are in a committed relationship?

- Anyone can act on their personal lust and have sex when they feel like it. How might waiting to have sex show deeper feelings for someone?

- Have you heard of "revenge sex" (having sex with someone to get back at another person or make them jealous)? What are your thoughts on this?

- How do you feel when you hear about someone you know having casual hook-up sex?

- You are going to have friends who have different ideas about sex. How can you talk about your views without being rude or judgmental?

## Additional Resources:

"'Are You Having Sex?'" from Educate and Empower Kids
Listed in this article are a few less awkward ways to approach the topic of sexual activity with your teen.

"I Was a Teenage SLUT" from Educate and Empower Kids
This article tells a cautionary tale of poor self-esteem and social pressure, and what to do to avoid situations like this.

# 27.
# The Double Standard & Derogatory Terms

 **DOUBLE STANDARD:** *A rule or standard that is applied differently and/ or unfairly to a person or distinct groups of people.*

Although certain positive strides have been made to improve the quality of life for women and men all over the world, some double standards and derogatory terms–often aimed at women–still remain. As our teenagers grow more independent throughout their middle school and high school years, it's important to be straightforward about the realities of these cultural stereotypes and double standards.

Explain that, when it comes down to the heart of the matter, the purpose of derogatory terms is to embarrass and dehumanize people. Open a discussion about the various reasons why people would want to treat others that way. Sometimes people find it easier to write someone off as a chick, babe, or doll rather than to get to know them and see them as a woman. Challenge your child to avoid derogatory terms and question double standards in our culture.

## Start the Conversation

Start by talking about what a derogatory term is. Ask your teen for specific derogatory or slang terms they've heard for girls, boys, or sex, and what's meant by them. Decide if you should bring up any they haven't mentioned. Ask them why they think there are so many more negative terms for women than men. Tell your child how you feel when you hear these words. Discuss ways they can cope with these terms when the words are directed at them. Explain that one of the purposes of derogatory terms is to humiliate and dehumanize people. Open a discussion about the various reasons why people would want to treat others that way.

Talk about misogyny and misandry (see glossary): what they are, where they may have come from, and what your child can do to stand up to these negative ideas and behaviors. Discuss slut-shaming (see glossary), which is focusing on a girl's promiscuous sexual behavior whether she is actually promiscuous or not.

Discuss some of the double standards that occur in our culture. Be sure to talk about ones that are unfair to both women, men, and other social groups. One classic, sexual double standard is that men don't get bad sexual reputations for promiscuity, but women do for the same behavior and actions. Another double standard is that men and boys are typically praised for sexual contacts while women are controlled sexually through judgment, shame, and humiliation. Discuss reasons why these and other double standards exist. Talk about the double standards that existed in your teenage years.

## Questions for Your Child

○ Our culture still has double standards when it comes to the sexual behavior of men, women, girls, and boys. Why do you think they exist?

○ Why do we sometimes hold women to a higher standard of morality? Are there other standards in our society that we expect men to do better?

○ Why do double standards exist?

○ Have you observed any double standards in your home? At church? At school?

○ What can you do to change or stand up to double standards?

○ Have you ever been called a derogatory name or term? How did you handle it?

○ Have you ever used derogatory names or terms?

○ How does slut-shaming impact a girl's humanity and dignity?

○ What are the strengths that men have? What are strengths that women have? Why do we need both men's and women's strengths?

○ You will know people throughout your life who have different ideas and standards of morality. What can you do to ensure that you treat each individual with respect and see them in a positive light?

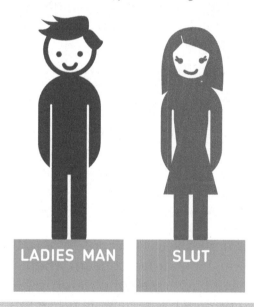

LADIES MAN    SLUT

## Additional Resources:

"Sex Talks for Daughters" from Media Savvy Moms, March 2020
This is a podcast featuring Educate and Empower Kids discussing what important sexual topics you should talk about with your daughters.

"Porn Addiction Is Not Just a 'Boys' Problem' Anymore" from Educate and Empower Kids
Pornography is a rampant problem for all ages and all people; this article goes through a few ways to help your daughters if they've grown addicted to this dangerous substance.

"Translating Slang for Parents" from Educate and Empower Kids
This article contains a list of commonly used internet slang to help parents understand what certain phrases or acronyms mean.

"Parent Dictionary: Search Engine Terms" from Educate and Empower Kids
This article also goes through a list of terms and abbreviations for inappropriate or popular language used on the internet, way too many of which are derogatory terms for women and their anatomy.

# 28.
# Sex Under the Influence

This is a very relevant topic for teenagers because experimenting with drugs and alcohol is so widespread. Talking about drugs and alcohol now will help your teen think more critically and make decisions for themself before they're in a situation that could get out of hand.

 **UNDER THE INFLUENCE:** *Being physically affected by alcohol or drugs.*

Spend time discussing consent and how a person cannot give consent when they have had any alcohol or drugs (whether they have willingly taken the drugs or been given them without their permission). Share your wisdom with your child. If you have had negative experiences because of you or someone else making poor decisions during drug or alcohol use, now is the time to share what the consequences were.

## Start the Conversation

Explain that people who are drunk, high, or under the influence of a substance do things that they wouldn't otherwise do. Alcohol and drugs impair judgment, physical coordination, and natural inhibitions. Alcohol and drug use often open the door to many risky behaviors.

Help your teen have a plan for avoiding drinking in various scenarios (at a friend's house, during a sleepover, while at a party, etc.). Discuss different options for getting out of a situation where they don't feel comfortable. Review how alcohol and drugs influence decision-making. Talk about "Consent" in lesson #10 as needed.

Open a discussion about the emotional fallout from making bad decisions while under the influence of a drug or alcohol. Finally, teach your child to have a safety plan when alcohol, drugs, or other dangerous substances are present in their social engagements. It is not enough to simply keep themself safe; if they are with friends, they should look out for their friends as well.

Consider having a code word that your child can text you. It may not even have to come from their phone number. Agree on how you will help them. For example, when you get their message, you will pick them up, no questions asked.

Non-consensual sex is rape, and one cannot consent if one has been drinking or is otherwise incapacitated.

## Questions for Your Child

- How does someone who is drunk, high, or under the influence of drugs behave?

- People drink alcohol or take drugs for a number or reasons (to let their inhibitions down, to have fun, to relax, to escape their problems, to look "cool," etc.). Have you seen someone do things when drunk or high that are out of character?

- Why is it a bad idea to drink or take drugs around people you don't know or fully trust?

- Can a person give consent or receive consent while they're drinking or doing drugs?

- What is meant by the term "date rape drug"? What effect do these have on people?

- If you are at a party or other social situation, why should you never leave your drink unattended?

- If you do drink alcohol or try drugs of your own choice and someone takes advantage of you sexually, are you at fault? (NO! You cannot give consent while under the influence. Even if you choose to drink or do drugs, assault is NEVER your fault!)

### Sample Scenario

Share the following scenario to your teen:

You're at a party and see a girl who is clearly drunk and not in control of herself. Two guys are gradually cornering her, getting closer and beginning to touch her casually. As you watch, they become more aggressive, touching and grabbing her. She doesn't seem to totally comprehend what's going on, but she does weakly try to move away from them. They continue in their actions anyway. Are you going to have the courage to speak up? What will you say?

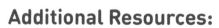

## Additional Resources:

"Talking With My Children About Rape" from Educate and Empower Kids
It's important not only to talk to your kids about rape, but to talk to them early enough that the information can come from someone who loves them.

"3 Practical Suggestions to End Victim Blaming" from Educate and Empower Kids
A start to ending rape culture is to end victim blaming, and this article goes through helpful and practical ways to do that.

# 29.
# STDs & STIs

Please avoid any thought of "my child would never" when approaching this or any other topic in this book. We must teach our kids the most correct principles we can, then they must exercise their agency from there. Our kids must be educated about the stark realities of sexually transmitted infections and diseases. These are powerful illnesses that can have physical repercussions throughout a person's entire life.

The Centers for Disease Control and Prevention (CDC) estimates that there are 25 million new cases of sexually transmitted infections and diseases each year and $16 billion in associated medical costs. Almost half of these new cases occur in young people ages 15-24. The number of STD cases is skyrocketing among teen boys and girls. Be sure to cover the topics of infection transmission, prevention, and testing. Speak with a doctor or health professional if you or your teens need further help.

## Start the Conversation

First, ask your teen which sexually transmitted diseases they have heard about or have been taught about at school or elsewhere. Discuss specific STDs and STIs such as herpes, chlamydia, gonorrhea, syphilis, hepatitis, AIDS, HIV, and pubic lice (these and other helpful terms can be found in the glossary). Point out that some STDs last a lifetime. These include HIV, herpes, HPV, and hepatitis B.

Explain how STDs can be passed through oral, anal, and vaginal sex. Emphasize that STD rates among teens has increased profoundly because many teens wrongly believe that infection and disease can only occur through vaginal sex. Explain that a person can get an STD the first time they have oral, anal, or vaginal sex. Be frank and tell your child that sometimes teenagers and adults lie about their

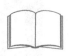 **STD & STI:**
*Abbreviations that refer to sexually transmitted diseases or infections. These are illnesses that are communicable through sexual behaviors, including, but not limited to, intercourse.*

sexual history. This is why getting tested is so important before one gets married and after having unprotected sex.

Share your ideas and values about prevention. Explain that the most effective means of prevention is abstinence followed by monogamy. However, the next best thing is to use a condom during every sexual encounter where semen, vaginal secretions, or blood may be present.

Remind your child that waiting until they are in a committed relationship to have sex will not only protect your child from certain emotional baggage, it can also protect them against unwanted pregnancy and STDs.

## Questions for Your Child

- Do you know how various STDs and STIs affect the body?
- Which STDs can be cured with treatment? Which ones cannot be cured with treatment?
- How can you avoid STDs and STIs?
- Some people don't like the feel of a condom. Is your own or your partner's sexual pleasure through unprotected sex more important than your health?
- If one of your friends confides in you that they have had an STI or STD, how could you compassionately respond?
- What would you do if you suspect you have an STD?

> People who refuse to use condoms do not deserve to have sex with anyone but other people who refuse to use condoms.

## Additional Resources:

"Sexually Transmitted Disease Surveillance" from the Centers for Disease Control and Prevention (CDC)
The CDC provides more information, data, and statistics on STDs and how to prevent them.

"Adolescents and Young Adults" from the CDC
This page provides links to videos and other resources about how to talk to your child about these topics and gives more information on STDs.

# 30.
# Birth Control

Even if you think your child is not having sex or would never have sex out of a committed relationship, it's important that both your sons and daughters know what birth control methods are available. Use your personal values as you guide this conversation. Discuss what you feel is most important for your teenager to know and understand.

**CONTRACEPTIVE:**
*A method, device, or medication that works to prevent pregnancy. Another name for birth control.*

Teen birth rates have been slowly declining over the past 20 years. However, we are not out of the woods. With many young women having legal abortions and using emergency contraception such as the morning-after pill, it's clear that although there may be some decrease in kids having vaginal sex, there are still too many teenage girls getting pregnant.

Teach your child the sad facts of teen pregnancy. According to the Centers for Disease Control (CDC), children of teenage mothers are more likely to have lower school achievement, drop out of high school, have more health problems, be incarcerated at some time during adolescence, give birth as a teenager, and face unemployment as a young adult.

Don't shy away from talking about abortion, which is not pregnancy prevention. It is a method of terminating a pregnancy. Talk about the alternative: legal adoption. If you have a friend or loved one who has faced making the decision of keeping a baby or giving it up for adoption, share what you know with your child.

## Start the Conversation
Use the glossary to talk about different forms of birth control/contraceptives, such as abstinence, pills, patches, implants, shots, IUDs, diaphragms, condoms, and the rhythm method. Examine the effectiveness of each method. Remind your child that abstinence is the only 100% effective birth control method. Explain that abstinence or condoms are necessary to prevent STDs.

**Educating your children on various forms of birth control will NOT make them have sex any earlier. It will simply protect them from unwanted pregnancy and/or disease.**

Have a discussion about the benefits of starting a family under the best circumstances, with two loving, committed parents. Share your experience and knowledge about having a baby when one is emotionally and financially ready to have a child. Talk about what it would have been like—or what it was like—under economically or emotionally difficult circumstances. Ask your child to share their views on what the best circumstances are to bring a child into the world.

Talk about what your family would do if your son got someone pregnant or if your daughter became pregnant before a committed relationship or marriage. Discuss possible situations where birth control may come under debate. Ask your child what they would do if their partner tried to pressure them to have sex without using a condom or some other form of birth control.

## Questions for Your Child

- ○ What are some different forms of birth control? Is birth control the responsibility of the woman, the man, or both partners?

- ○ Why might some people avoid birth control or condoms despite how easy they are to get and use? Can you think of any reason to not use a condom or other birth control and risk an unwanted pregnancy?

- ○ How should a woman decide what birth control is right for her?

Q Why are there still debates about birth control when it's so easy to get and can usually be gotten for free?

Q What are some less effective or ineffective methods of birth control? (Pulling out before ejaculation, the rhythm method, etc.)

Q What do you think of teen birth rate statistics in light of so many available birth control methods?

Q Are there any positive aspects to being an unmarried, teenage parent?

Q What are the best circumstances under which to have a family? What are the benefits to each family member in waiting to have a baby until these are in place?

Q What should you do if you or your partner gets pregnant before you are married or in a serious, committed relationship?

## Sample Dialogue

Share the following joke with your child:

> **Parent:** What do you call people who use the "rhythm method"?
>
> **Child:** I don't know. What do you call them?
>
> **Parent:** Mommies and Daddies.

## Additional Resources:

"4 Easy Steps to Creating Healthy Communication About Sexual Intimacy" from Educate and Empower Kids
The best way to help your kids stay safe sexually, physically, and emotionally is to have healthy relationships with solid communication between parent and child. This article can help give some tips on how to establish those.

"7 Steps to Take to Establish Yourself as an Approachable Parent" from Educate and Empower Kids
This article goes through some helpful tips on how to let your kids know you are trustworthy and approachable and that they can come to you about anything.

"Holding Family Meetings: A Necessity for Our Busy Families" from Educate and Empower Kids
Knowing how to hold a family meeting where all can share and relate to one another is one of the best ways to open those lines of communication, and this article can help you do that.

"From Awkward to Awesome: Talking to Your Kids About Sexual Intimacy" from Educate and Empower Kids
Talking to your kids about sexual intimacy, including STDs or contraception, doesn't need to be awkward. It can be a helpful, meaningful experience. Learn what you need to talk about and how to talk about sex with your younger and older kids.

# TOPIC CARDS

# CUT OUT THESE TOPIC CARDS TO HELP YOU START TALKING!
## Post one on your refrigerator to remind yourself,
## or to let your kids know, of the upcoming discussion.

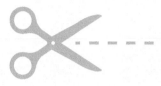

## 1. THE PHYSICAL SIDE OF RELATIONSHIPS

- Is there a natural progression of affection in a relationship?
- What are some different ways that people show affection?
- Do you decide the next step in your relationship or does your partner?
- Does biology or social experience determine how people feel about sex?

## 2. SEX

- What is sex?
- What "counts" as sex?
- What types of sex are there?

## 3. EMOTIONAL INTIMACY

- The best sex has strong emotional connection.
- Do you need emotional intimacy to have sex?
- Is it okay to have sex purely for physical satisfaction?
- Can you have true intimacy without a physical relationship?

## 4. SEX MEANS DIFFERENT THINGS TO BOYS & GIRLS

- What does sex mean to you?
- Is it a myth that boys only want to have sex for physical gratification?
- Many people, especially females equate having sex

## 5. POSITIVE ASPECTS OF SEX

- It fosters emotional bonding/closeness/unity.
- It's fun.
- It can be a connection on the most human/innate level possible.
- It feels awesome.

## 6. PHYSICAL RESPONSES TO SEX

- What happens when a male is sexually aroused?
- What happens when a female is sexually aroused?
- Physical responses to sex are individual

## 7. ORGASM

- What is an orgasm?
- Do you need to have an orgasm for sex to be fullfilling?
- Men and women achieve orgasm differently.

## 8. RELATIONSHIP BOUNDARIES

- At what age is it okay to have sex?
- At what point in a relationship is it okay to have sex?
- Is it okay to stop once you've started?
- Should you be in a committed relationship before having sex?

## 9. FIRST TIME

- What are your expectations for your first time?
- How will you feel/react if it's different?
- How will you know if you are ready?

## 10. CONSENT

- How do you know he or she really means yes?
- What is rape?
- Is it okay to stop once you've started?
- What is rape culture?

## 11. CREATING A HEALTHY RELATIONSHIP

- Learning to communicate
- Cultivating respect and dignity
- Developing healthy ideas of intimacy

## 12. ABUSIVE RELATIONSHIPS

- Abuse can be emotional, mental, physical and/or sexual
- Why are some people abusive to others?
- How do you stop abuse?

## 13. SELF-WORTH & SEX

- How does your self-worth affect your decisions about intimacy?
- A person who loves & respects themselves will not demean others.
- Will sex empower or diminish you?

## 14. LIKING YOURSELF

- You are entitled to great relationships.
- You can make great decisions.
- You are entitled to emotional intimacy.

## 15. BODY IMAGE & SEX

- How does body image affect our inherent sense of value?
- How do you feel about the way you look?
- Do you create relationships based on people's looks?
- Will your body image affect your sex life?

## 16. BEING MEDIA SAVVY

- What does the media teach us about sex and relationships?
- How can you create your own ideas about sex and relationships in a culture of powerful messages?
- Do the people you see in media look like the people in your everyday life?

## 17. PORNOGRAPHY

- What is pornography?
- When is the last time you saw something pornographic?
- Why is pornography damaging to individuals, relationships, and society?

## 18. MASTURBATION

- What constitues masturbation?
- Do you feel that masturbation is healthy? Why or why not?
- Are there consequences to making it a habit?

## 19. SHAME & GUILT

- Why do some people think sex is "bad" or "dirty"?
- Why are we curious about sex?
- What situations could cause shame or guilt about sex?

## 20. SEXTING & SOCIAL MEDIA

- What is sexting?
- What should you do if you get sext messages or images?
- Why do people feel they can say things on social media that they would never say face to face?

## 21. SEXUAL CONVERSATIONS

- Do you think it's appropriate for an adult other than your parents to discuss sex with you?
- When it comes to sex, what are kids talking about?
- Are these conversations helpful?

## 22. SEXUAL IDENTIFICATION

- It is individual.
- Understand that sexuality can be fluid, changing over time; it can also be constant.
- Your sexuality is an intregal part of you but does not define who you are.
- What are some factors that can influence your sexuality?

## 23. UNWANTED SEXUAL ATTENTION

- What constitutes unwanted sexual attention?
- Telling the other person to stop is your right.
- Some sexual attentions or behaviors are illegal.

## 24. HOW PREDATORS GROOM KIDS

- What does it mean for a predator to groom?
- Predators are often people the teenager knows.
- Predators may use "innocent" and "affectionate" touch to desensitize and build trust.
- Predators can be your peers and other teenagers.

## 25. MONOGAMY VS MULTIPLE PARTNERS

- What is monogamy?

- What are some emotional and spiritual benefits of monogamy?

- What are some health benefits of monogamy?

- Are there risks to having multiple partners?

## 26. SEX IN A COMMITTED RELATIONSHIP VS HOOK UP SEX

- How do you think sex in a committed relationship differs from hook up sex?

- Why do people in a committed relationship have sex?

- Why do people have hook up sex?

## 27. THE DOUBLE STANDARD & DEROGATORY SLANG TERMS

- What are derogatory terms used for men? For women?

- How do you feel when you hear them?

- What is slut-shaming and how does it impact women?

- What is the sexual double standard that exists in our culture?

- Derogatory terms are meant to humiliate and dehumanize.

## 28. SEX UNDER THE INFLUENCE

- How does alcohol or drugs affect your behavior?

- Alcohol and drugs impair your ability to consent or receive consent.

- What would sex under the influence be like compared to sober sex?

## 29. STDs & STIs

- Do you know the names and symptoms of STDs and STIs?

- Some STDs and STIs last a lifetime.

- Prevention includes regular condom use and abstinence, followed by monogamy, and

## 30. BIRTH CONTROL

- What are various methods of birth control?

- Having a baby when you're emotionally and financially ready is positive and extraordinary.

- The only 100% effective birth control method is abstinence.

# GLOSSARY

*The following terms have been included to assist you as you prepare and hold discussions with your children regarding healthy sexuality and intimacy. The definitions are not intended for the child; rather, they are meant to clarify the concepts and terms for the adult. Some terms may not be appropriate for your child, given their age, circumstances, or your own family culture and values. Use your judgment to determine which terminology best meets your individual needs.*

**Abortion:** An abortion is a procedure to end a pregnancy. It uses medicine and/or surgery to remove the embryo or fetus and placenta from the uterus.

**Abstinence:** The practice of not doing or having something that is wanted or enjoyable; the practice of abstaining from something.

**Abuse:** The improper usage or treatment of another person or entity, often to unfairly gain power and/or other benefit in the relationship.

**Affection:** A feeling of liking or caring for something or someone. A type of love that surpasses general goodwill.

**AIDS:** A sexually transmitted or bloodborne viral infection that causes immune deficiency.

**Anal Sex:** A form of intercourse that generally involves the insertion and thrusting of the erect penis into the anus and rectum for sexual pleasure.

**Anus:** The external opening of the rectum, composed of two sphincters which control the exit of feces from the body.

**Appropriate:** Suitable, proper, or fitting for a particular purpose, person, or circumstance.

**Arousal (in regards to sexual activities):** The physical and emotional response to sexual desire during or in anticipation of sexual activity. In men, this results in an erection. In women, arousal results in vaginal lubrication (wetness), engorgement of the external genitals (clitoris and labia), and enlargement of the vagina.

**Birth Control:** The practice of preventing unwanted pregnancies, especially by use of contraception. See also IUD, condom, contraceptive implant, and the pill.

**Birth Control Shot:** Commonly referred to as the birth control shot, Depo-Provera® is an injectable form of birth control. This contraceptive option is a shot that contains the hormone progesterone and is given on a regular schedule.

**Bisexual:** A sexual orientation in which one is attracted to both males and females.

**Body Image:** An individual's feelings regarding their own physical appearance, attractiveness, and/or sexuality. These feelings and opinions are often influenced by other people and media sources.

**Bodily Integrity:** The personal belief that our bodies, while crucial to our understanding of who we are, do not in themselves solely define our worth. The knowledge that our bodies are the storehouse of our humanity, and the sense that we esteem our bodies and we treat them accordingly. It is also defined as the right to autonomy and self-determination over one's own body.

**Boundaries:** The personal limits or guidelines that an individual forms in order to clearly identify what are reasonable and safe behaviors for others to engage in around him or her.

**Bowel Movement:** Also known as defecation, a bowel movement is the final act of digestion by which waste is eliminated from the body via the anus.

**Breasts:** Breasts contain mammary glands, which create the breast milk used to feed infants. Women develop breasts on their upper torso during puberty.

**Child:** A term often used in reference to individuals who are under the age of 18. This overlaps with the term "teen."

**Circumcision:** The surgical removal of foreskin from a baby's penis.

**Chlamydia:** A common sexually transmitted infection caused by the bacteria chlamydia trachomatis. It can affect the eyes and may cause damage to a woman's reproductive system.

**Clitoris:** A female sex organ visible at the front juncture of the labia minora above the opening of the urethra. The clitoris is the female's most sensitive erogenous zone.

**Condom:** A thin rubber covering that a man wears on his penis during sex in order to prevent a woman from becoming pregnant and/or to help prevent the spread of diseases.

**Consent:** Clear agreement or permission to do something. Consent must be given freely, without force or intimidation, while the person is fully conscious and cognizant of their present situation.

**Contraceptive:** A method, device, or medication that works to prevent pregnancy. Another name for birth control. See birth control, IUD, condom, or diaphragm.

**Contraceptive Implant:** A long-term birth control option for women. A contraceptive implant is a flexible plastic rod about the size of a matchstick that is placed under the skin of the upper arm.

**Curiosity:** The desire to learn or know more about something or someone.

**Date Rape:** A rape that is committed by someone with a person they have gone on a date with. The perpetrator uses physical force, psychological intimidation, and/or drugs or alcohol to force the victim to have sex either against their will or in a state in which they cannot give clear consent.

**Degrade:** To treat with contempt or disrespect.

**Demean:** To cause a severe loss in dignity or respect in another person.

**Derogatory:** An adjective that implies severe criticism or loss of respect.

**Diaphragm (Contraceptive):** A cervical barrier type of birth control made of a soft latex or silicone dome with a spring molded into the rim. The spring creates a seal against the walls of the vagina, preventing semen, including sperm, from entering the fallopian tubes.

**Domestic Abuse/Domestic Violence:** A pattern of abusive behavior in any relationship that is used by one partner to gain and/or maintain power and control over another in a domestic setting. It can be physical, sexual, emotional, economic, and/or psychological actions or threats of actions that harm another person. (From the Department of Justice.)

**Double Standard:** A rule or standard that is applied differently and/or unfairly to a person or distinct groups of people.

**Egg Cell/Ovum:** The female reproductive cell, which, when fertilized by sperm, will eventually grow into an infant.

**Ejaculation:** When a man reaches orgasm and semen is expelled from the penis.

**Emotion:** An emotion is a feeling such as happiness, love, fear, sadness, or anger, which can be caused by the situation that you are in or the people you are with.

**Emotional Abuse:** A form of abuse in which another person is subjected to behavior that can result in psychological trauma. Emotional abuse often occurs within relationships where there is a power imbalance.

**Emotional Intimacy:** A form of intimacy that displays a degree of closeness which focuses more on the emotional over the physical aspects of a relationship.

**Epididymal Hypertension:** A condition that results from prolonged sexual arousal in human males in which fluid congestion in the testicles occurs, often accompanied by testicular pain. The condition is temporary, and is also referred to as "blue balls."

**Erection:** When the penis becomes engorged/enlarged with blood, often as a result of sexual arousal.

**Explicit:** In reference to sexual content, "sexually explicit" is meant to signify that the content with such a warning will portray sexual content openly and clearly to the viewers.

**Extortion:** To obtain something through force or threats, particularly sex or money.

**Family:** A group consisting of parents and children living together in a household. The definition of family is constantly evolving, and every person can define family in a different way to encompass the relationships they share with people in their life. Over time one's family will change as one's life changes and the importance of family values and rituals deepen.

**Female Arousal:** The physiological responses to sexual desire during or in anticipation of sexual activity in women. This includes vaginal lubrication (wetness), engorgement of the external genitals (clitoris and labia), enlargement of the vagina, and dilation of the pupils.

**Fertilize:** The successful union between an egg (ovum) and a sperm, which normally occurs within the second portion of the fallopian tube, also known as the ampulla. The result of fertilization is a zygote (fertilized egg).

**Forced Affection:** Pressuring or forcing a child to give a hug, kiss, or any other form of physical affection when they do not have the desire to do so.

**Foreskin:** The fold of skin which covers the head (the glans) of the penis. Also called the prepuce.

**Friend:** Someone with whom a person has a relationship of mutual affection and is typically closer than an associate or acquaintance.

**Gay:** A slang term used to describe people who are sexually attracted to members of the same sex. The term "lesbian" is generally used when talking about women who are attracted to other women. Originally, the word "gay" meant "carefree"; its connection to sexual orientation developed during the latter half of the 20th century.

**Gender:** Masculinity and femininity are differentiated through a range of characteristics known as "gender." However, use of this term may include biological sex (being male or female), social roles based upon biological sex, and/or one's subjective experience and understanding of their own gender identity.

**Gender Role:** The commonly perceived pattern of masculine or feminine behavior as defined by an individual's culture and/or upbringing.

**Gender Stereotypes:** A generalized thought or understanding applied to either males or females (or other gender identities) that may or may not correspond with reality. "Men don't cry" or "women are weak" are examples of inaccurate gender stereotypes.

**Gestation:** The period of time when a person or animal is developing inside its mother's womb preparing to be born.

**Gonorrhea:** A sexually transmitted disease that affects both males and females, usually the rectum, throat, and/or urethra. It can also infect the cervix in females.

**Grooming (Predatory):** To prepare/train and/or desensitize someone, usually a child, with the intent of committing a sexual offense and/or harm.

**Healthy Sexuality:** Having the ability to express one's sexuality in ways that contribute positively to one's own self-esteem and relationships. Healthy sexuality includes approaching sexual relationships and interactions with mutual agreement and dignity. It must include mutual respect and a lack of fear, shame, or guilt and never include coercion or violence.

**Hepatitis B:** Hepatitis B (HBV) is an incurable disease which is most commonly spread through exposure to infected bodily fluids via unclean needles, unscreened blood, and/or sexual content. It can manifest as acute or chronic. The acute form can resolve itself in less than six months, but it will often turn chronic. The chronic form can persist in the body for a lifetime and lead to a number of serious illnesses including cirrhosis and liver cancer. The younger a person is exposed to HBV, the more likely it will become chronic.

**Hepatitis C:** Similarly transmitted to Hepatitis B, Hepatitis C attacks the liver. Though most individuals with Hepatitis C are asymptomatic, individuals who do develop symptoms typically show signs of yellowing skin and eyes, fatigue, and/or nausea.

**Herpes:** A series of diseases of the skin caused by the herpes virus which cause sores and inflammation of the skin. Type 1 viruses will manifest as cold sores on the lips or nose, while the type 2 viruses are sexually transmitted and specifically known as genital herpes. This causes painful sores on the genital area.

**Heterosexual:** Sexual orientation in which one is attracted to members of the opposite sex (males are attracted to females; females are attracted to males). See also, straight.

**HIV:** HIV (human immunodeficiency virus) is a virus that attacks the body's immune system. If not treated, it will turn into AIDS.

It is incurable and will persist in the body for life. It is spread through infected bodily fluids and sexual contact.

**Homosexual:** Sexual orientation in which one is attracted to members of the same sex (males are attracted to males; females are attracted to females). See also gay or lesbian.

**Hookup Sex:** A form of casual sex in which sexual activity takes place outside the context of a committed relationship. The sex may be a one-time event, or an ongoing arrangement. In either case, the focus is generally on the physical enjoyment of sexual activity without an emotional involvement or commitment.

**HPV:** Human papillomavirus. It is the most common STD in the United States and can cause genital warts or cancer in about 10% of those infected. Anyone over age 10 can receive the vaccine for HPV.

**Hymen:** A membrane that partially closes the opening of the vagina and whose presence is traditionally taken to be a mark of virginity. However, it can often be broken before a woman has sex simply by being active, and sometimes it is not present at all.

**Hyper-sexualized:** To make extremely sexual; to emphasize the sexuality of. Often seen in media.

**Instinct:** An inherent response or inclination toward a particular behavior. An action or reaction that is performed without being based on prior experience.

**Intercourse:** Sexual activity, also known as coitus or copulation, that most commonly understood to refer to the insertion of the penis into the vagina (vaginal sex). It should be noted that there are a wide range of various sexual activities and the boundaries of what constitutes sexual intercourse are still under debate. See also, sex.

**Intersex:** An umbrella term used to refer to the rare phenomenom of an individual born with some mixture of both male and female reproductive anatomy. This can be very obvious with visibly deformed or underdeveloped reproductive organs, to something as subtle as alterations in the xy chromosomes. It's also possible for signs of intersex to not develop until later in life.

**Intimacy:** Generally, a feeling or form of significant closeness. There are four types of intimacy: physical intimacy (sensual proximity or touching), emotional intimacy (close connection resulting from trust and love), cognitive or intellectual intimacy (resulting from honest exchange of thoughts and ideas), and experiential intimacy (a connection that occurs while working together). Emotional and physical intimacy are often associated with sexual relationships, while intellectual and experiential intimacy are not. However, people can engage in a sexual experience that is devoid of intmacy.

**IUD:** A small, T-shaped device that is placed in the uterus to prevent pregnancy.

**Labia:** The inner and outer folds of the vulva on both sides of the vagina.

**Lesbian:** A word used to describe women who are sexually attracted to other women.

**Lice (Pubic):** A sexually transmitted sucking louse infesting the pubic region of the human body.

**Love:** A wide range of emotional interpersonal connections, feelings, and attitudes. Common forms include kinship or familial love, friendship, divine love (as demonstrated through worship), and sexual or romantic love. In biological terms, love is the attraction and bonding that functions to unite human beings and facilitate the social and sexual continuation of the species.

**Masturbation:** Self-stimulation of the genitals in order to produce sexual arousal, pleasure, and/or orgasm.

**Media Literacy:** The ability to study, interpret, and create messages in various media such as books, social media posts, online ads, movies, etc. It also includes understanding how to navigate being online, what to avoid, and what information to share and/or keep private.

**Menstrual Cycle:** The egg is released from ovaries through the fallopian tube into the uterus. Each month, a lining of blood and tissue build up in the uterus. When the egg is not fertilized, this lining is no longer needed and is shed from the body through the vagina. The cycle is roughly 28 days, but can vary between individuals. The bleeding lasts around 2-7 days. The menstrual cycle may be accompanied by cramping, breast tenderness, and emotional sensitivity.

**Menstrual Period:** A discharging of blood, secretions, and tissue debris from the uterus as it sheds its thickened lining (endometrium) approximately once per month in females who've reached a fertile age. This does not occur during pregnancy.

**Misandry:** Like misogyny, it is the hatred, aversion, hostility, or dislike of men or boys. Similarly, it also can appear in a single individual, or may also be manifest in broad cultural trends.

**Misogyny:** The hatred, aversion, hostility, or dislike of women or girls. Misogyny can appear in a single individual, or may also be manifest in broad cultural trends that undermine women's autonomy and value.

**Molestation:** Aggressive and persistent harassment, either psychological or physical, of a sexual manner.

**Monogamy:** A relationship in which a person has one partner at any one time.

**Nipples:** The circular, somewhat conical structure of tissue on the breast. The skin of the nipple and its surrounding areola are often several shades darker than that of the surrounding breast tissue. In women, the nipple delivers breast milk to infants.

**Nocturnal Emissions:** A spontaneous orgasm that occurs during sleep. Nocturnal emissions can occur in both males (ejaculation) and females (lubrication of the vagina). The term "wet dream" is often used to describe male nocturnal emissions.

**Non-binary/Genderqueer:** Non-binary or genderqueer is an umbrella term for gender identities that are neither male nor female—identities that are outside the gender binary. Non-binary identities fall under the transgender umbrella, since non-binary people typically identify with a gender that is different from their assigned sex.

**Nudity:** The state of not wearing any clothing. Full nudity denotes a complete absence of clothing, while partial nudity is a more ambiguous term, denoting the presence of an indeterminate amount of clothing.

**Oral Sex:** Sexual activity that involves stimulation of the genitals through the use of another person's mouth.

**Orgasm:** The rhythmic muscular contractions in the pelvic region that occur as a result of sexual stimulation, arousal, and activity during the sexual response cycle. Orgasms are characterized by a sudden release of built-up sexual tension and the resulting sexual pleasure.

**Penis:** The external, male sexual organ comprised of the shaft, foreskin, glans penis, and meatus. The penis contains the urethra, through which both urine and semen travel to exit the body.

**Perception:** A way of regarding, understanding, or interpreting something; a mental impression.

**Period:** The beginning of the menstrual cycle.

**Physical Abuse:** The improper physical treatment of another person with the intent to cause bodily harm, pain, or other suffering. Physical abuse is often employed to unfairly gain power or other benefit in the relationship.

**The Pill:** An oral contraceptive for women containing the hormones estrogen and progesterone or progesterone alone. This prevents ovulation, fertilization, or implantation of a fertilized ovum, causing temporary infertility.

**Polyamory:** The practice of engaging in multiple romantic (and typically sexual) relationships, with the agreement of all the people involved.

**Pornography:** The portrayal of explicit sexual content for the purpose of causing sexual arousal. In it, sex and bodies are commodified for the purpose of making a financial profit. It can be created in a variety of media contexts, including videos, photos, animation, books, and magazines. Its most lucrative means of distribution is through the internet. The industry that creates pornography is a sophisticated, corporatized, billion-dollar business.

**Positive Self-Talk:** Anything said to oneself for encouragement or motivation, such as phrases or mantras; also, one's ongoing internal conversation with oneself, like a running commentary, which influences how one feels and behaves.

**(Sexual) Predator:** Someone who seeks to obtain sexual contact/ pleasure from another through predatory and/or abusive behavior. The term is often used to describe the deceptive and coercive methods used by people who commit sex crimes with a victim.

**Pregnancy:** The common term used for gestation in humans. During pregnancy, the embryo or fetus grows and develops inside a woman's uterus.

**Premature Ejaculation:** When a man regularly reaches orgasm, during which semen is expelled from the penis, prior to or within one minute of the initiation of sexual activity.

**Priapism:** The technical term of a condition in which the erect penis does not return to flaccidity within four hours, despite the absence of physical or psychological sexual stimulation.

**Private:** Belonging to or for the use of a specific individual. Private and privacy denote a state of being alone, solitary, individual, exclusive, secret, personal, hidden, and confidential.

**Psychological Abuse:** A form of abuse where the abuser regularly uses a range of actions or words with the intent to manipulate, weaken, or confuse a person's thoughts. This distorts the victim's sense of self and harms their mental wellbeing. Psychological abuse often occurs within relationships in which there is a power imbalance.

**Puberty:** A period or process through which children reach sexual maturity. Once a person has reached puberty, their body is capable of sexual reproduction.

**Public:** Belonging to or for the use of all people in a specific area, or all people as a whole. Something that is public is common, shared, collective, communal, and widespread.

**Queer:** A historically derogatory term against people who were homosexual, that has been reclaimed by the LGBTQ+ community. It is also an umbrella term for sexual and gender minorities who are not heterosexual.

**Rape:** A sex crime in which the perpetrator forces another person to have sexual intercourse against their will and without consent. Rape often occurs through the threat or actuality of violence against the victim.

**Rape Culture:** A culture in which rape is pervasive and, to an extent, normalized due to cultural and societal attitudes towards gender and sexuality. Behaviors that facilitate rape culture include victim blaming, sexual objectification, and denial regarding sexual violence.

**Relationship:** The state of being connected, united, or related to another person.

**Rhythm Method:** A method of avoiding pregnancy by restricting sexual intercourse to the times of a woman's menstrual cycle when ovulation and conception are least likely to occur. Because it can be difficult to predict ovulation, the effectiveness of the rhythm method is on average just 75–87%.

**Romantic Love:** A form of love that denotes intimacy and a strong desire for emotional connection with another person to whom one is generally also sexually attracted.

**Scrotum:** The pouch of skin underneath the penis that contains the testicles.

**Self-Worth/Self-Esteem:** An individual's overall emotional evaluation of their own worth. Self-worth is both a judgment of the self and an attitude toward the self. More generally, the term is used to describe a confidence in one's own value or abilities.

**Semen:** The male reproductive fluid, which contains spermatozoa in suspension. Semen exits the penis through ejaculation.

**Serial Monogamy:** A mating system in which a man or woman can only form a long-term, committed relationship (such as marriage) with one partner at a time. Should the relationship dissolve, the individual may go on to form another relationship, but only after the first relationship has ceased.

**Sex (Sexual Intercourse):** Sexual activity, also known as coitus or copulation, which is most commonly understood to refer to the insertion of the penis into the vagina (vaginal sex). It should be noted that there are a wide range of various sexual activities and the boundaries of what constitutes sexual intercourse are still under debate. See also, intercourse.

**Sexting:** The sending or distribution of sexually explicit images, messages, or other material via phones, email, or instant messaging.

**Sexual Abuse:** The improper sexual usage or treatment of another person, often to unfairly gain power or other benefit in the relationship. In instances of sexual abuse, undesired sexual behaviors are forced upon one person by another.

**Sexual Assault:** A term often used in legal contexts to refer to sexual violence. Sexual assault occurs when there is any non-consensual sexual contact or violence. Examples include rape, groping, forced kissing, child sexual abuse, and sexual torture.

**Sexual Harassment:** Harassment involving unwanted sexual advances or obscene remarks. Sexual harassment can be a form of sexual coercion as well as an undesired sexual proposition, including the promise of reward in exchange for sexual favors.

**Sexual Identification:** How one thinks of oneself in terms of whom one is romantically or sexually attracted to.

**Shame:** The painful feeling arising from the consciousness of something dishonorable, improper, ridiculous, etc., done by oneself or another.

**Slut-shaming:** The act of criticizing, attacking, or shaming a woman for her real or presumed sexual activity, or for behaving in ways that someone thinks are associated with her real or presumed sexual activity.

**Sperm:** The male reproductive cell, consisting of a head, midpiece, and tail. The head contains the genetic material, while the tail is used to propel the sperm as it travels towards the egg.

**Spontaneous Erection:** A penile erection that occurs as an automatic response to a variety of stimuli, some of which is sexual and some of which is physiological.

**STD:** An abbreviation that refers to sexually transmitted diseases, many of which persist in the body for life. These are illnesses that are communicable through sexual behaviors, including intercourse. Some of these illnesses can also be transmitted through contact with various bodily fluids.

**STI:** An abbreviation that refers to sexually transmitted infections. These are illnesses that are communicable through sexual behaviors, including intercourse. Some of these illnesses can be transmitted through blood contact. Not all STI's lead to a disease and become an STD.

**Straight:** A slang term for heterosexuality, a sexual orientation in which one is attracted to members of the opposite sex (males are attracted to females; females are attracted to males). See also, heterosexual.

**Syphilis:** Syphilis is an infection typically spread through sexual contact. It is a chronic, contagious, usually venereal and often congenital disease. If left untreated, syphilis can produce chancres, rashes, and systemic lesions in a clinical course with three stages continued over many years.

**Test Touch:** Seemingly innocent touches by a predator or offender, such as a pat on the back or a squeeze on the arm, that are meant to normalize kids to being in physical contact with the predator. Test touches can quickly progress from these innocent touches to more dangerous and damaging ones.

**Testicles:** The male gonad, which is located inside the scrotum beneath the penis. The testicles are responsible for the production of sperm and androgens, primarily testosterone.

**Transgender:** A condition or state in which one's physical sex does not match one's perceived gender identity. A transgender individual may have been assigned a sex at birth based on their genitals, but feel that this assignation is false or incomplete. They also may be someone who does not wish to be identified by conventional gender roles and instead combines or moves between them (often referred to as gender-fluid).

**Uncomfortable:** Feeling or causing discomfort or unease; disquieting.

**Under the Influence:** Being physically affected by alcohol or drugs.

**Urethra:** The tube that connects the urinary bladder to the urinary meatus (the orifice through which the urine exits the urethra tube). In males, the urethra runs down the penis and opens at the end of the penis. In females, the urethra is internal and opens between the clitoris and the vagina.

**Urination:** The process through which urine is released from the urinary bladder to travel down the urethra and exit the body at the urinary meatus.

**Uterus:** A major reproductive sex organ in the female body. The uterus is located in the lower half of the torso, just above the vagina. It is the site in which offspring are conceived and in which they gestate during pregnancy.

**Vagina:** The muscular tube leading from the external genitals to the cervix of the uterus in women. During sexual intercourse, the penis can be inserted into the vagina. During childbirth, the infant exits the uterus through the vagina.

**Vaginal Discharge/Secretions:** Vaginal discharge is the umbrella term for the clear/milky white fluid that secretes from the vagina daily. This discharge is the means by which the vagina keeps itself clean by discharging cells and debris. When a woman is sexually aroused, she will see an increase in this secretion as a means of preparing the vagina for sex.

**Vaginal Sex:** A form of sexual intercourse in which the penis is inserted into the vagina.

**Vaginismus:** A medical condition in which a woman experiences pain from any form of vaginal penetration, including sexual intercourse, the use of tampons or menstrual cups, and/or gynecological examinations.

**Victim:** A person who is harmed, injured, or killed as the result of an accident or crime.

**Virgin:** A person, male or female, who has never engaged in sexual intercourse.

**Vulva:** The parts of the female sexual organs that are on the outside of the body.

**Wet Dreams:** A slang term for nocturnal emissions. A nocturnal emission is a spontaneous orgasm that occurs during sleep. Nocturnal emissions can occur in both males (ejaculation) and females (lubrication of the vagina).

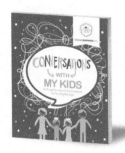

### *Conversations With My Kids: 30 Essential Family Discussions for the Digital Age*

Parenting in the digital age has never been tougher. The world is changing faster than we can keep up with! It seems like there's always a new toy or device at every turn. With all this new tech, comes new information and new dangers. Our kids are exploring world issues and personal questions you and I didn't face at their age. Conversations With My Kids gives you the words and handy discussion questions to have meaningful talks about 30 very timely topics.

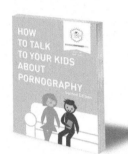

### *How to Talk to Your Kids About Pornography: 2nd Edition*

Never before has it been so easy to talk with your children or teens about this tough topic. With smartphones and tablets everywhere, our kids are engaged in one of the most incredible social experiments ever conceived in the history of mankind. Within this alarming experiment, our children are becoming entrenched in an increasingly pornified culture. Take the time now to protect and prepare your family. Whether they are 6 or 16, you will have worthwhile, relevant discussions that will educate and prepare your family. Also available in Spanish.

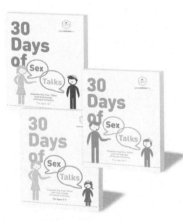

### *30 Days of Sex Talks Empowering Your Child with Knowledge of Sexual Intimacy*

Written by parents and reviewed by professionals, 30 Days of Sex Talks makes it simple for you and your child to talk about the mechanics of sex, emotional intimacy, healthy and abusive relationships, and so much more. We've broken down "the talk" into 30 uncomplicated "chats" to make it simple for you to engage in these critical conversations with your children. Remember, talking to your kids about healthy sexuality doesn't have to be awkward! It can be very empowering for you and your kids.

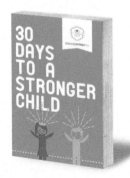

### *30 Days to a Stronger Child*

As our families face an uncertain future, there are skills and qualities we must help our children develop in order for them to grow resilient, strong, and successful. That's why we've given you an engaging, straightforward way to teach the vital concepts of physical health, emotional strength, social skills, spiritual balance, and intellectual growth to your children. We've included activities, discussions, and questions that will empower you to raise a stronger, more exceptional child.

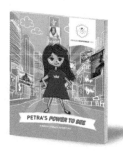

### Petra's Power to See: A Media Literacy Adventure

We are surrounded by messages (media)—most of them are beautiful! Some inspire us to learn and grow, but some messages are empty and unhealthy. Join Petra and her dad as they venture into the city to learn about the powerful media messages all around us. They come face to face with clear and hidden messages in different media such as advertising, social media, and fake news. Petra and her dad will teach you what media is, how it affects us, and how to make wise choices when using media.

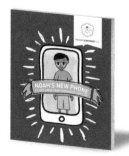

### Noah's New Phone: A Story About Using Technology for Good

When Noah gets a smartphone for his birthday, he quickly realizes the power he holds in his hands. He becomes aware of its power to do good and inspire positive change as well as its negative and hurtful capacity. A great read-together book, Noah's New Phone also includes a handy workbook to reinforce important elements of the story like choices, safety, healthy boundaries and the huge potential within technology.

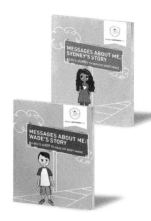

### Messages About Me: Sydney's Story: A Girl's Journey to Healthy Body Image

### Messages About Me: Wade's Story: A Boy's Quest for Healthy Body Image

Our kids receive hundreds, possibly thousands of messages every day from friends, family members, acquaintances, advertisements, social media, TV, and elsewhere. Join Sydney and Wade on their individual journeys as they first struggle and then, with the help of parents and a good friend, come to understand they are happy to be themselves and are truly beautiful the way they are.

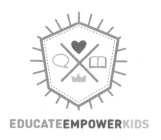

**EDUCATEEMPOWERKIDS**

# IF YOU ENJOYED THIS BOOK,
# PLEASE LEAVE A POSITIVE REVIEW ON
# AMAZON.COM

Subscribe to our websites for
exclusive offers and information,

www.educateempowerkids.org

Be sure to check out our accompanying video series for this book
at educateempowerkids.org

To view or download the additional resources listed at the end of
each lesson, please follow the link in this QR code.

Made in the USA
Las Vegas, NV
15 May 2024

89957949R00077